"Weight loss is irrelevant to improving your health."

- Stanford Owen, M.D.

The PrescriptFit® Medical Nutrition Therapy plan is designed for those desiring diet strategy as an aid to medical management of disease. It is not intended to replace physician management and should be used in conjunction with physician treatment and oversight. Consultation and follow-up with your physician is strongly advised prior to, and concurrent with, using the PrescriptFit MNT plan.

Claims of medical benefit have not been evaluated by the U.S. Food and Drug Administration (FDA). Nutritional recommendations and guidelines of the PrescriptFit MNT plan are compatible with most professional guidelines and recommendations.

Those with sensitivity to egg or milk products should use PrescriptFit products with caution as they contain egg white protein and milk solids.

Questions regarding PrescriptFit products or the PrescriptFit plan can be addressed at www.drdiet.com or by contacting us at 1-888-460-6286.

Published by:
drdietmedia, LLC
3300 15th St.
Gulfport, MS 39501
888-460-6286

*Medical Writing and Editing/Graphic Design and Layout:*
Kathi L. Whitman, In Credible English®, Salt Lake City, UT

ISBN 978-0-9760290-5-2

Printed in the United States of America
     10  9  8  7  6  5  4  3  2  1

©2017 Stanford A. Owen, MD

# PRESCRIPTFIT®
MEDICAL NUTRITION THERAPY ■ ■ ■ ■ ■ ■ ■ ■

# FOREWORD

There are so many things to like about PrescriptFit Medical Nutrition Therapy (MNT), from the layout, graphics, and easy-to-read text to the "stories" – case histories – that make the lessons of this book come alive. Also, the approach is not "one size fits all" but instead personalizes the MNT strategy, allowing patients to enter the program at different phases according to their profile/needs.

By far the greatest achievement in this book is the way Dr. Owen links the comorbidities to weight gain and emphasizes disease severity as the driver of how intense the approach should be. To my knowledge, there is no rival book in the realm of popular "diet books" that links weight loss so persuasively to health improvement. Dr. Owen's many years of experience in medical weight loss comes across as does the fact that he genuinely cares for his patients.

Dr. Owen has so much hands-on experience — over 25 years treating diabetes and metabolic-related illness, following patients through different phases of their lives, and helping them manage relapse when life events derail their wellness plans. This sort of experience is not common, and the book and PrescriptFit plan are valuable additions to popular weight loss literature.

Donna H. Ryan MD,
Professor EmeritaPennington Biomedical Research Center
Baton Rouge, LA

### About Dr. Ryan

*Donna Ryan is the Charter Medical Director of Pennington Biomedical Research Center, the largest nutrition research center in the world. She is a Past President of the International Obesity Society and serves as Associate Editor in Chief of the journal, Obesity.*

*Dr. Ryan co-chairs the panel to revise the NIH-supported evidence-based Guidelines on the Evaluation and Management of Overweight and Obesity in Adults. Her scholarly activities include authorship of more than 170 original publications and 45 books, chapters and reviews, primarily in the field of obesity. She has served the scientific community as a reviewer and advisor in many capacities including the following: NSF Medical R&D Expenditures Workshop 2006; National Dairy Council Review Team for Children's Hospital Oakland Research Institute, 2006; Chair, Data Safety Monitoring Board (DSMB), NIH Grant, "Safety and Efficacy of Low and High Carbohydrate Diets," 2002-2008, Member DSMB for EARLY Studies 2010- present and reviewer for European Union Innovative Medicines Iniatiative, 2011-12. Dr. Ryan has served as a scientific advisor and/or consultant to Abbott, Knoll, Procter and Gamble, Novartis, TAP Pharmaceuticals, Slim Fast, Solvay, Weight Watchers, Alere Wellbeing, Nutrisystem, Vivus, Arena, Sanofi-Aventis, Ajinomoto, Merck, Takeda, Vivus, Eisai, Arena, Novo-Nordisk and Scientific Intake.*

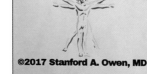

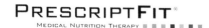

**PRESCRIPTFIT**
MEDICAL NUTRITION THERAPY ▪ ▪ ▪ ▪ ▪ ▪ ▪

©2017 Stanford A. Owen, MD

# PREFACE

**Weight Loss is Irrelevant!** Reducing symptoms, improving metabolism, and controlling diabetes. Note that none of these reference weight loss.

I started prescribing Medical Nutrition Therapy (MNT) in the early 1980s and was so drawn to the treatment results that by 1990, I decided to pursue MNT full time. I did not know why, in 1980, patients healed by diet strategies, by using nutrition supplements, and by exercising: they just did—and did so profoundly and in hours and days, not months and years. How could removal of certain "toxic" foods and addition of other "perfect" engineered food improve symptoms and physical findings SO dramatically and SO quickly?

**I became compelled to know WHY?**

Since the 1990s mountains of nutrition, obesity, and endocrine scientific studies state over and over again that only 5% of weight loss is necessary to achieve meaningful clinical benefit. REALLY? 5%? In other words, a 350-pound woman would only need to lose 15-20 pounds to medically improve while still 200 pounds overweight? Why also do bariatric surgeons, more often than not, send their massively obese patients home from the hospital a day after bariatric surgery discontinued off of all diabetic medication, never to have it reinstated **because their blood sugar improved on DAY 1?**

**Because it's the diet, not the weight!** Now, most of my patients lose weight. Many lose considerable weight, yet the most improvement of symptoms or disease measure is noted in the first 4-8 weeks. WHY?

The discovery of leptin and scores of additional cytokine proteins produced by fat cells solved the mystery of benefits I've witnessed in my MNT patients for the past 30 years. These cytokine proteins govern all aspects of metabolism, inflammation, and insulin resistance and respond to your last meal as well as your total body fat stores.

**Today, I no longer wonder why patients improve.** Fat cells become "angry" and produce toxic cytokines when overfed, old, and misguided by diseased genes. Angry fat cells cause disease. Angry fat cells change mood and behavior. Cytokine proteins mediate that "anger."

The coming years of my practice will see expanded knowledge of recent discoveries. We will better understand the brain and behavior. We may further learn to improve metabolism with medication and/or nutrition.

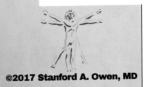

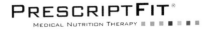

PRESCRIPTFIT®
MEDICAL NUTRITION THERAPY ■ ■ ■ ■ ■ ■ ■

We may even crack the code of addictive behavior that plagues society from overeating to drug and alcohol abuse.

**For every patient I see, the primary concerns involve whether or not a diet plan is safe, if it produces desired results, and can the patient see measurable change.** It is important that people can register benefits to diet and behavior change each and every time they follow the plan. It is equally important that the plan can be used in everyday situations and by the entire family. Above all, it must be simple, enjoyable, and reasonably affordable.

**PrescriptFit® Medical Nutrition Therapy (MNT) achieves these goals.**

**This book offers you a usable, readable way to learn about and begin practicing PrescriptFit strategies.** Section A covers the science behind PrescriptFit. Section B offers step-by-step guidance for each food phase, including cooking tips and links to recipes and shopping lists. Section C details how MNT helps reduce symptoms in a variety of common medical conditions and gives you ways to track your symptoms with your healthcare provider throughout the Plan. The PrescriptFit Calendar (available at www.drdiet.com) makes it easy to incorporate PrescriptFit strategies into your lifestyle right away. **Above all, I want PrescriptFit to help you live a longer and richer life.**

**Questions, comments?** Please contact us at 888-460-6286, or visit our Web site: www.drdiet.com.

*[signature]*

**PRESCRIPTFIT**®
MEDICAL NUTRITION THERAPY ▪ ▪ ▪ ▪ ▪ ▪

©2017 Stanford A. Owen, MD

# Contents

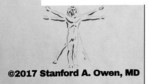

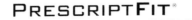

PRESCRIPTFIT®

MEDICAL NUTRITION THERAPY ▪ ▪ ▪ ▪ ▪ ▪ ▪

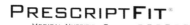

PRESCRIPTFIT
MEDICAL NUTRITION THERAPY ▪ ▪ ▪ ▪ ▪ ▪ ▪

©2017 Stanford A. Owen, MD

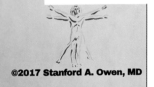

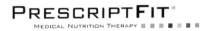

PRESCRIPTFIT®
MEDICAL NUTRITION THERAPY ■ ■ ■ ■ ■ ■ ■

# SECTION A

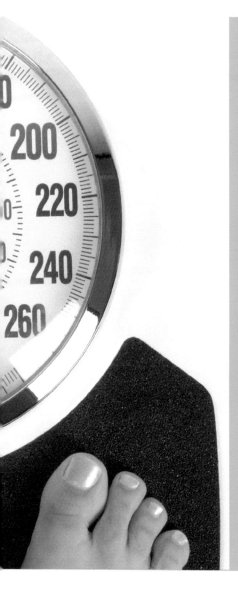

Taking Control –
Making
PrescriptFit
Work for You

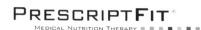

**PRESCRIPTFIT** ®
MEDICAL NUTRITION THERAPY ▪ ▪ ▪ ▪ ▪ ▪ ▪ ▪

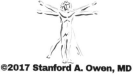

# TABLE OF CONTENTS

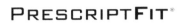

©2017 Stanford A. Owen, MD

# SECTION A: TAKING CONTROL — MAKING PrescriptFit WORK FOR You

PrescriptFit® Medical Nutrition Therapy (MNT), is a unique dietary strategy for controlling disease and improving symptoms. The strategy relies on these key concepts:

> **The impact of amino acids (the building blocks of protein in our bodies) on wellness** — As we age and become more overweight, our bodies produce chemicals called "cytokines" at levels that cause illness. **Branched-chain and essential amino acids,** given in a precise formula, appear to improve cytokine balance and metabolism, reduce inflammation, and alleviate illness symptoms.

*Essential amino acids must be acquired from one's diet. They cannot be manufactured by the body from other proteins.*

> **Positive reinforcement tends to change behavior** — Because PrescriptFit stresses regularly measuring results, you quickly see improvement. When you record that you're taking fewer pain medications, sleeping through the night more often, or experiencing less indigestion, it's much easier to stick with what's working.

> **Real solutions need to be "real-world" solutions** — Each of us struggles with time, money, family, and work constraints that make changing eating habits difficult. PrescriptFit offers a simple, flexible, cost-effective, and enjoyable, long-term solution.

> **There's more to diet success than just following a "plan"** — This approach helps you get ready for success with tips for changing your environment and habits surrounding eating as well as for talking with your healthcare provider about PrescriptFit Plan.

*PrescriptFit stresses:*

- *How to reduce symptoms of illness through better nutrition*

- *Why flexibility in a diet plan is critical to long-term success*

- *How getting ready to change your eating habits is the most important "insurance" you can have for making that plan a success*

- *Why collaborating with your health-care provider and family will make seeing and feeling results more likely*

## PRESCRIPTFIT®
MEDICAL NUTRITION THERAPY ■ ■ ■ ■ ■ ■ ■ ■

**©2017 Stanford A. Owen, MD**

# CHAPTER 1:
# WHAT IS PRESCRIPTFIT?

PrescriptFit is a type of Medical Nutrition Therapy (MNT) designed to help people control a variety of chronic (and sometimes life-threatening) illnesses through diet strategies. MNT is a process you follow to understand what foods cause you damage and what foods do not as well as what foods can actually heal your underlying metabolism and cellular function. Our entire goal is to help you heal and feel better. Weight loss is a side effect.

PrescriptFit uses recent medical findings about how our bodies process what we eat to solve a number of both disease- and weight-related problems.

Two key terms you will want to remember when discussing PrescriptFit with a qualified healthcare provider are cytokines and branched-chain amino acids.

## BALANCING CYTOKINES AND BRANCHED-CHAIN AMINO ACIDS FOR WELLNESS

In the field of nutritional science, we have learned some fascinating lessons in the last decade or two. **One of those lessons is that cytokines — proteins produced by fat tissue — orchestrate how most of our body's organs work.** These cytokines are essential to metabolism and preserve immune and organ function; however, when they become out of balance, disease in multiple organs occurs. This imbalance can contribute independently to heart disease, arthritis, depression, and injury to nerve cells and blood vessels — all findings in patients with type 2 diabetes.

# PRESCRIPTFIT™
MEDICAL NUTRITION THERAPY ▮ ▮ ▮ ▮ ▮ ▮ ▮

# CHAPTER 1: WHAT IS PRESCRIPTFIT?

Discovered in the 1990s, the first of these cytokines, leptin, governs fat storage, fertility, hunger, sugar metabolism, and the immune system. Scores of cytokines discovered since leptin have equally diverse functions.

Cytokine overproduction is influenced by:

> Being overweight or obese (especially with a large belly)

> Failing to exercise regularly

*Although we've known there was a link between obesity and disease for centuries, only recently have we discovered what appears to be the source of that link — cytokines.*

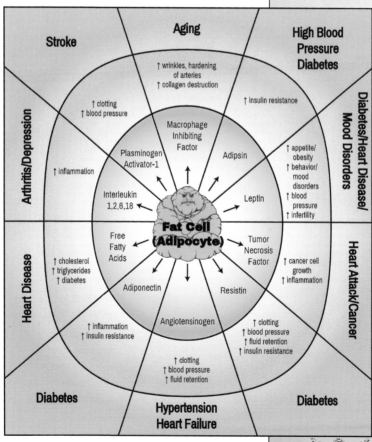

# ~ SECTION A: TAKING CONTROL... ~

*Foods we eat without problems when we're kids may cause serious health problems in adulthood. Why? Because age and fat cell distribution accelerate cytokine overproduction, often triggering development of diseases we're at risk for based on family history.*

*Cytokine imbalance and its impact on feelings of hunger, satiety, cravings, and appetite may explain why some people, previously slim and trim as teenagers, only now look down at large abdomens; others may have struggled with obesity their entire lives.*

> Overeating and consuming high-fat, high-carbohydrate foods

> Aging

> Having an inherited likelihood of having certain diseases such as diabetes or hypertension

**Cytokines and Behavior** — Perhaps more important than the immune, metabolic, or cardiovascular effects of cytokines are their effects on nerve cells in areas of the brain that affect our behavior. These areas of the brain control:

> Appetite

> Energy expenditure (both voluntary exercise and involuntary movement)

> Motivation

> Hunger and cravings

> Feelings of fullness

Cytokines are produced in response to your last meal as well as to your total body fat stores. They affect brain function related to feeding, explaining why one person is "stuffed" after a moderate meal while the next person returns for third servings without discomfort.

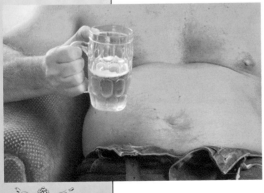

This link between behavior and cytokines explains why foods impact us differently and how we think about eating as we age.

**PRESCRIPTFIT**
MEDICAL NUTRITION THERAPY ▪ ▪ ▪ ▪ ▪ ▪

# ⇜ CHAPTER 1: WHAT IS PRESCRIPTFIT? ⇝

Why, for example, does a person who was previously active and vibrant, now feels sluggish and unproductive? The answer — cytokines are adversely affecting the brain AND metabolism.

**Branched-chain Amino Acids (BCAAs): an Antidote for Out-of-Balance Cytokines** — The other important lesson learned from recent nutritional research is that there is a way to control cytokine imbalance through proteins called "branched-chain amino acids." Amino acids are the building blocks of protein in our bodies; we don't produce those amino acids essential to this process — they must come from our diet. The term, "branched-chain amino acids," refers to the molecular structure of certain amino acids linked to reducing inflammation, improving metabolism, and fostering growth in childhood.

One of the most important findings has been that amino acids play a key role in telling our bodies how to best use insulin — a hormone secreted by the pancreas that helps the body use blood glucose (blood sugar) for energy or store it for future use in the form of glycogen in liver or muscle cells. More and more people today suffer from something referred to as "insulin resistance," which occurs when the body cells "resist" using normal or even elevated insulin secreted by the pancreas. The result is a back-up of insulin in the bloodstream, which is related to an imbalance in the fats stored in the blood — causing unhealthy cholesterol levels

*When combined with structured food plans, specific types of protein, called branched-chain amino acids, assist in normalizing this cytokine imbalance. Branched-chain amino acids added to your diet improve appetite control and energy.*

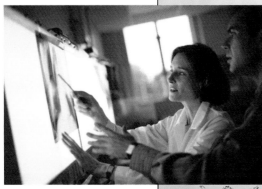

(increased triglycerides, decreased HDL [good] cholesterol). These unhealthy cholesterol levels dramatically increase a person's risk of heart disease.

While obesity and lack of regular exercise can lead to insulin resistance, important new research indicates that amino acids also play a vital role in "signaling" the insulin secreted by the pancreas to more effectively metabolize fat cells. This metabolic "signaling" is key to preventing and reducing insulin resistance and improving metabolism.

Amino acids promote the release of a gut hormone "glucagon-like peptide-1" or "GLP-1," which improves insulin and metabolism. Medications that promote the release of GLP-1 act in a very similar way as the amino acids in PrescriptFit.

### LINKING BCAAS AND CYTOKINES WITH PRESCRIPTFIT

When fat cells are "fed" balanced nutrition that contains branched-chain and essential amino acids, cytokine balance improves.

**Amino Acids and Medical Treatment** — A number of scientific research studies have shown that amino acids play a significant role in treating many of today's most common illnesses and physical problems. Most notably, the *American Journal of Cardiology* published a variety of articles that documented key research in the role of amino acids in counteracting chronic diseases, such as heart failure, type 2 diabetes and insulin resistance, and liver cirrhosis. Other research has linked depression and other affective disorders (such as anxiety, ADHD, bipolar disorder, and others) in part to

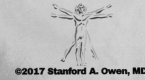

**PRESCRIPTFIT**
MEDICAL NUTRITION THERAPY ▪ ▪ ▪ ▪ ▪ ▪ ▪

inflammation in the brain that may result from cytokine imbalance.

What this research tells us is that there is an apparent link between getting cytokines in balance and reducing symptoms of various physical and mental disorders.

SECTION B WILL HELP YOU EASILY WORK WITH STRUCTURED FOOD PHASES, WHICH ARE KEY TO PRESCRIPTFIT.

Using sequentially added Food Phases with amino acids helps you optimize illness treatment in new ways. For example, if you suffer from acid reflux as well as fatigue, high blood pressure and diabetes, your symptoms should all decrease significantly following the first couple of Food Phases. Then, when you add nuts (Food Phase 6), you notice that your acid reflux returns while fatigue, blood pressure, and sugar control remain perfect. When you add pork and beef (Food Phases 9 and 10), you start experiencing fatigue and your blood pressure goes up due to the effects of saturated fat, while blood sugar remains normal. Your diabetes-related blood sugar may not elevate until you add dairy products and starchy foods (Food Phases 12 and 13).

What you've learned is exactly how the foods you eat impact your symptoms AND perhaps what quantities you can have and not feel deprived. You discover that the same "damaging" food group may be well tolerated with limited exposure, so that you can regulate those damaging delights in "splurge" meals scattered throughout the month. By being sensitive to symptoms (fatigue), following signs (e.g., swelling), and checking objective measures (e.g., blood pressure or blood sugar level), patients learn to avoid harm inflicted by specific food groups.

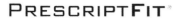

# ~ SECTION A: TAKING CONTROL... ~

**Amino Acids and the PrescriptFit™ Medical Nutrition Therapy Plan** — Modifying food intake while using the essential amino acid supplements in the PrescriptFit Medical Nutrition Therapy (MNT) Plan normalizes fat-cell cytokine production, improving disease symptoms and health measurements. PrescriptFit amino acid supplements are formulated using egg white and nonfat milk solids and are fortified with a unique formula of *(micronized)* branched-chain and essential amino acids: leucine, isoleucine, valine, lysine, and histidine.

The PrescriptFit MNT Plan is a three-step approach to lifelong diet and wellness:

1. **Step One:** Medical Treatment. You will use amino acids as medical treatment for disease symptoms. Without fail, this total nutrition solution (nothing else is required besides a multivitamin) is the foundation for feeling better and losing weight.

2. **Step Two:** Healing and Education. By "phasing" in food groups, the Plan promotes healing and self education about calories and nutrition. When we focus on individual food groups for a specific time, we learn how best to prepare, eat, and combine different foods with amino acid supplements for optimum health and enjoyment.

3. **Step Three:** Splurging. PrescriptFit MNT makes "splurge" meals a regular part of a healthy approach to eating. NO ONE can diet forever. PrescriptFit recognizes our need to splurge; this is the diet that teaches you to manage and enjoy social eating.

Overall, the plan includes 13 Food Phases representing all major food groups. You will not be

Medical Treatment

PrescriptFit®

Splurging

Healing & Education

**PRESCRIPTFIT**
MEDICAL NUTRITION THERAPY ■ ■ ■ ■ ■ ■ ■

deprived of any food. Each Food Phase is built on the experience and results of each previous Food Phase. PrescriptFit allows you to design a healthy eating style to fit any taste, budget, or cultural preference.

Food Phase 1 uses food supplements containing branched-chain amino acids as total nutrition. These amino acid-containing supplements are continued with every Food Phase to normalize sugar and fat metabolism. The products also provide fullness and satiety to control appetite and cravings. By balancing cytokine production from fat cells, branched-chain amino acids influence activity of disease or behaviors deemed unrelated until now.

| PRESCRIPTFIT DAILY DOSING | |
|---|---|
| For Best Results | 6-8 doses (scoops) |
| To Maintain Your Success | 5+ doses (scoops) |
| Maximum Allowed (for strenuous exercise training programs) | 20 doses (scoops) |

Specific food categories, beginning with those with the least fat and carbohydrate count, progressing to those with the highest fat and carbohydrate content, are added to the PrescriptFit amino acid products sequentially. Each subsequent Food Phase teaches food science, nutrition, and culinary arts for that category.

## PROVING SUCCESS — MEASURING SYMPTOM AND DISEASE RESPONSE

The Prescript Fit™ Medical Nutrition Therapy (MNT) Plan recognizes disease response to food and measures that response as a function of the diet plan. You get positive reinforcement when your symptoms improve or you gain control over your illness.

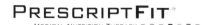

**PRESCRIPTFIT**
MEDICAL NUTRITION THERAPY ▪ ▪ ▪ ▪ ▪ ▪ ▪

# ~ SECTION A: TAKING CONTROL... ~

*Most people with diabetes have some degree of sugar addiction. Every patient 100 pounds overweight is food addicted.*

Similarly, you experience negative reinforcement when there is a relapse of signs or symptoms after adding new Food Phases, failing to take the recommended doses of amino acid product, or splurging too often. When this happens, you simply return to Food Phase I and repeat the 13-phase Plan. Even the three-day/Food-Phase Plan will register improvement in weight and health measures.

The MNT Plan uses symptom and disease questionnaires to measure change in your health and wellness at regular intervals. This element of PrescriptFit helps to educate and motivate you for long-term health improvement. Medical conditions and symptoms improve measurably and quickly using MNT. Work with your healthcare provider to use the Symptom/ Disease Questionnaires in section C to measure improvement on a regular basis. Some medical tests should be measured at provider-defined intervals. When improvements are noted, continue the Prescript Fit™ Plan indefinitely, just as you would continue to use any medication that alleviates illness symptoms.

*Scores of different cytokine proteins have been recently identified, each with its unique effects on different organs.*

Many different and unrelated diseases improve with MNT. It is well known that diabetes or hypertension will improve with diet intervention. Heart disease and depression may also improve with MNT since cytokines from fat tissue may contribute independently to each condition. Therefore, a particular type or amount of food may contribute to different conditions simultaneously by the same fat cell-produced cytokine.

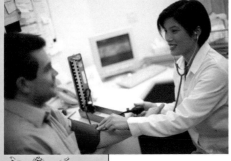

PRESCRIPTFIT®
MEDICAL NUTRITION THERAPY ■ ■ ■ ■ ■ ■ ■

# CHAPTER 1: WHAT IS PRESCRIPTFIT?

## UNDERSTANDING FOOD ADDICTION

*Are you "addicted" to foods that keep you overweight?*

*Does this "food addiction" cause you to suffer from diabetes, hypertension, heart disease, joint or back pain, sleep apnea, fatigue, and exhaustion?*

*Are you ostracized and excluded socially because of your weight?*

*Why is it so hard to stay on the weight-loss plan your healthcare provider recommends even though you know your health is at stake?*

Understanding how your brain processes the messages it receives from the food you eat will help answer these challenging questions.

## FOOD ADDICTION AND YOUR BRAIN

**Do you have classic symptoms of "addiction"?** The circuits in your brain transmit messages about substances that bring us pleasurable experiences. Then, our brains chemically code those messages into a lasting feeling of reward. We reinforce these codes with repeated exposure to these substances plus the social or sensory associations we have with that pleasure experience. For example, you may meet your friends for coffee and donuts every Saturday morning at a nearby coffee shop. Your brain codes both the pleasure of eating those tasty treats along with the pleasure of laughing and talking with your good friends. The pleasure memory cannot be erased or replaced. If you avoid the addictive substance (that awesome latte and jelly roll), you may suffer psychological, emotional, and physical pain (withdrawal), which can lead to binging.

*Taken faithfully, like a medication, these amino acid food products become a tool to aid in dietary compliance and lower food addiction feelings.*

*Some animals demonstrate signs of physical withdrawal and even epileptic seizures after becoming conditioned to and then quickly withdrawn from sugar.*

*Balancing brain chemicals that control appetite is an emerging science and art.*

**PRESCRIPTFIT**
MEDICAL NUTRITION THERAPY ▪ ▪ ▪ ▪ ▪ ▪ ▪

# ⌁ Section A: Taking Control... ⌁

We now know that many of the neural pathways involved in overeating behaviors are the same ones that are triggered for those addicted to alcohol or drugs. Recent research using brain imaging found that people who were overweight or obese who ate meals made up of processed foods high in sugars and carbohydrates experienced increased hunger and cravings between meals because of the areas of their brains that were stimulated by those foods. (Lennerz, Alsop, Holsen, et. al., 2013)

Too often, society treats someone who is addicted to something as having a character flaw, as needing to be ostracized, ignored, or locked away. This is wrong; addiction is very much a chemical problem! Aggressive approaches are mandatory to break this cycle; food addiction is very, very powerful and, as opposed to drug addiction, is often unrecognized by the lay and professional community.

### Food Addiction and Diabetes: A Vicious Cycle

Virtually every person with type 2 diabetes and pre-diabetes is food addicted. Why? Because the insulin resist-ance that causes these disorders "lives" on the cell surface and prohibits energy (sugar) and protein (for repair) from entering the brain cells that tell you that you are full (satiation). In addition, your fat, liver, pancreas, and gut cells produce myriad hormones

**Insulin resistance makes you think you are hungry.**

**Cytokines increase hunger and cravings for carbs.**

**Carbs worsen insulin resistance.**

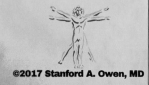

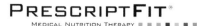

**PRESCRIPTFIT**®
MEDICAL NUTRITION THERAPY ▪ ▪ ▪ ▪ ▪ ▪ ▪

(cytokines) that decrease satiety (feeling of fullness) while increasing hunger, cravings (for carbs), and appetite (for social fun). Worse, those very foods someone with diabetes craves actually worsen insulin resistance, causing their brains to signal even more feelings of "starving." **What a vicious cycle!**

**Here's the good news.** A combination of lifestyle, food, and medication strategies will combat food addiction for those who are overweight, obese, and/or suffering from type 2 diabetes and other metabolic disorders. These strategies include:

> Engineered food to improve metabolism and brain chemistry

> Structured management of all food groups, especially Phases 9-13 (the addicting foods)

> Exercise

> A written tracking system for accountability

> Environmental cleanup (of food)

> Identification of familial and social habits and situations that undermine behavior change

> Treatments for mood disorders (depression, bipolar, anxiety)

> Removal of medications that contribute to obesity

> Medications for treating addiction behaviors

> Bariatric surgery

> Strong support from professionals (healthcare provider, addiction counselor)

FAMILIAL AND SOCIAL CONTRIBUTORS

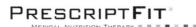

PRESCRIPT**FIT**
MEDICAL NUTRITION THERAPY ▪ ▪ ▪ ▪ ▪ ▪ ▪

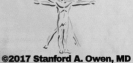

©2017 Stanford A. Owen, MD

# ~ Section A: Taking Control... ~

The "pushers" of the addicting products you are consuming are more than likely your spouse, your children, your parents, and your closest friends. They also include the social settings (e.g., the all-starch breakfast at scouting events, the pizza night each week with friends, etc.).

And what about the "pushers" who profit from our food purchases? The giant food companies with multibillion-dollar marketing teams stream images and sounds constantly into your television and computers, the magazines you read, and even ads that start showing up on your cell phone. Often, in my experience, those around you are completely unaware of how they undermine your health. Sadly, bariatric surgery is often the only way to survive in this environment of sabotage. Curiously, once the decision to undergo this kind of surgery is finalized, the patient can be criticized by those same loved ones for "lack of willpower"—a character flaw.

*Bariatric surgery can be lifesaving, but is often refused because of social stigma, If needed, bariatric surgery should never be refused because of prejudice that food addiction stems from a lack of willpower.*

## Food Addiction Therapy

Many options, thankfully, now exist to help with food addiction. All have benefits and risks, and each must be customized to the individual and carefully managed in concert with your healthcare provider. These options range from diet and exercise to bariatric (gastric bypass) surgery, which can cure type 2 diabetes and promises results no food program will achieve.

### Strategy #1 — Brain Detox

The PrescriptFit Food Phase Strategy utilizes addiction science in Phase 1 to protect and isolate the addicted brain.

Remove all decision-making from the equation. Eat only a shake, soup, or pudding for three, seven, or 14 days — even longer if successful. While this will work only for a short time to suppress addicting

PRESCRIPTFIT
MEDICAL NUTRITION THERAPY ▪ ▪ ▪ ▪ ▪ ▪

behavior, it may give the addicted brain time to heal and think more rationally. Think of this as similar to "residential" treatment for drug addiction. Most residential programs require at least a two-week, in-patient stay to "detox" the brain and body from the addicting drug while getting counseling. Most centers prefer one- to three-month stays to interrupt the behavior (and brain) patterns that support addiction. Many drug addicts, like food addicts, are actually malnourished by toxic or unbalanced nutrition. PrescriptFit products are "perfect food" from a healing perspective; they normalize the toxic cytokine environment that injures brain cells and contributes to addiction.

## Strategy #2 — Environmental Cleanup

Environmental Cleanup (EC) of addicting foods (Phases 9-13) is fundamental to "recovery." Put a heroin addict or alcoholic in the same environment after rehab, and relapse is all but assured. EC mandates the family and friends participate in the rehab. Discuss your addiction, ask their support, and, once you have it, hold them to it. Throw out all addicting food, whenever presented in the house, and confirm from the "pushers" that they, indeed, have committed to helping you with your addiction. Never back down. Doing this is tough! It takes practice.

## Strategy #3 — Exercise

Exercise creates natural endorphins that are chemically similar to morphine and heroin. Many successful food addicts become exercise addicts. Exercise reduces addicting and damaging cytokines and decreases insulin resistance from the muscle and brain cells. More is better when considering treating food addiction with exercise.

## Strategy #4 — Food Journaling

Accountability is key to all addiction programs. The

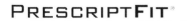

PRESCRIPTFIT
MEDICAL NUTRITION THERAPY ▪ ▪ ▪ ▪ ▪ ▪ ▪ ▪

©2017 Stanford A. Owen, MD

## ⁓ SECTION A: TAKING CONTROL... ⁓

most famous, Alcoholics Anonymous, is all about accountability. A 2008 Kaiser Permanente Center for Health Research study found that of 1,700 participants, those who kept food journals lost twice as much weight as those who did not. (Kaiser Permanente, 2008) Similarly, PrescriptFit user data confirm that patients are 85 percent more likely to achieve a positive outcome by simply keeping daily calendar data.

Use the PrescriptFit Calendar record system or the Calendar App to keep yourself accountable. The "Splurge" notation on the Calendar is your cue to addictive behavior. Most addiction overeating is with "Splurge" foods that combine carbohydrates with fats.

### Strategy #5 — Reducing Medications that Promote Food Addiction

Remove (when able) medications that tend to promote food addiction (and weight gain). The following describes each category; for a complete list with generic and brand name information, see appendix C. Be sure to discuss this strategy with your healthcare provider.

> **Cortisone (Prednisone)** — This steroid is used to treat inflammation. Cortisone steroids are administered orally, topically (skin creams), inhaled (asthma), and via injections (joint or epidural) and are usually prescribed/administered by physicians. Ask them for any and all other options. If you have been diagnosed with type 2 diabetes, all cortisone steroids will cause insulin resistance and make diabetes worse.

> **Psychiatric drugs** — These include antidepressant, anti-psychotic (both typical and the newer "atypical" medications), anti-epileptic, mood stabilizer, sedative, and pain medications.

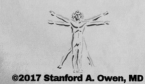

**PRESCRIPTFIT**®
MEDICAL NUTRITION THERAPY ▪ ▪ ▪ ▪ ▪ ▪ ▪

# ~ CHAPTER 1: WHAT IS PRESCRIPTFIT? ~

> **Antihistamines** — Yes, your favorite allergy medication or sleep aide may well contribute to food addiction and lower your metabolism. Even the so-called, "non-sedating" antihistamines available over the counter are contributory. Histamine is a primary brain neurotransmitter; suppressing certain histamine receptors slows metabolism and increases food-searching behavior.

> **Insulin** — Yes, the very drug used to treat some patients with type 2 diabetes actually causes increased appetite and fat cell growth. Removing insulin from the treatment equation, in my opinion, is crucial to long-term improvement in food control. Effective MNT, combined with medications listed in Strategy #6 below, frequently decrease symptoms, allowing patients to discontinue taking insulin (with healthcare provider approval/monitoring).

## Strategy #6 — Adding Medications that Diminish Food Addiction

The following describes each category of medications; detailed information about generic and brand names appears in appendix C. Be sure to discuss this strategy with your healthcare provider.

> **Insulin sensitizers** — If insulin causes increased appetite and weight gain, insulin sensitizers have the opposite effect. They allow foods to be metabolized properly and decrease the vicious cytokine cycle that addicts the brain to food. These include metformin, topiramate, H2 blockers (antacid pills), GLP-1 agonists, and certain appetite suppressants (e.g., phenteramine, locacertin).

PRESCRIPTFIT®
MEDICAL NUTRITION THERAPY ▪ ▪ ▪ ▪ ▪ ▪ ▪

# ~ Section A: Taking Control... ~

> **Antidepressants (dopamine agonists)** —
> These include bupropion, stimulants, and
> possibly some vitamins and minerals (e.g.,
> methylfolate, magnesium, chromium).

> **Opiate blockers** — Naltrexone blocks
> the effect of opiate-like endorphins on the
> addiction centers in the brain, especially
> when combined with dopamine-enhancing
> medications.

> **Amino acids (PrescriptFit products)**
> — Add these products to the meal when
> eating addicting foods. The amino acids
> are absorbed faster than sugar and
> partially block the negative effects of a
> high-fat, high-carb meal that provokes
> addicting cytokines.

## Strategy #7 — Bariatric Surgery

I present often at bariatric surgery meetings to
explain the role of PrescriptFit for enhancing
surgical outcomes. I note that nothing I can do
or prescribe is as powerful as bariatric surgery
in improving eating behavior, controlling type 2
diabetes, and producing weight loss with all the
medical benefits. The mechanisms explaining
why surgery is so successful are still being
unraveled, but they are clearly related to how the
gut and digestive hormones are involved in eating
behavior and metabolism. Most nutrition-related
disease resolves, including type 2 diabetes,
hypertension, lipid disorders, sleep apnea, fatty
liver, joint disease, and even depression.

Besides social and familial stigma, a primary
excuse I hear for not having this surgery is
cost. Morbid obesity is far costlier than any
bariatric procedure over a three-year period and
represents a massive cost-saving over decades
if you consider the costs associated with food,

*We are learning
much since the
widespread use of
bariatric surgery has
led to safer and better
outcomes.*

# PRESCRIPTFIT
MEDICAL NUTRITION THERAPY ▪ ▪ ▪ ▪ ▪ ▪ ▪

# ⟜ CHAPTER 1: WHAT IS PRESCRIPTFIT? ⟜

medication, and illness for someone who is obese, let alone the difference in quality of life, which is priceless. PrescriptFit products are used pre-operatively to improve metabolism leading up to surgery and to prevent complications (e.g., blood clots and infection). These products are used post-operatively to ensure perfect nutrition for healing and successful disease management.

In summary, PrescriptFit is a Medical Nutrition Therapy strategy. This strategy involves:

> **Using Engineered Food** — PrescriptFit shakes, soups, and puddings.

> **Adding Healthy Food to Your Diet** — Seafood, poultry, non-starchy vegetables, eggs, nuts, whole fruit, and even high-protein snack bars.

> **Managing Consumption of Animal Fats and Starches** —These animal fats and starches are toxic, but scrumptious and addicting. Managing is the right word. NOT AVOIDING OR REMOVING.

> **Treating Food Addiction** — PrescriptFit strategies may involve treating food addiction with medication as well as removing medications that cause weight gain and diabetes. Your healthcare provider is crucial in medication strategy. Finally, PrescriptFit strategy may even involve bariatric surgery to save lives and improve quality of life.

PrescriptFit is NOT a shake. It is NOT a diet plan. It is DIET STRATEGY.

# PRESCRIPTFIT
MEDICAL NUTRITION THERAPY ▪ ▪ ▪ ▪ ▪ ▪ ▪

# ∽ SECTION A: TAKING CONTROL... ∽

*Unlike other diets that promote weight loss with a side benefit of feeling better, PrescriptFit focuses on feeling better with an added bonus of losing weight.*

*As you progress on the PrescriptFit Plan, note:*

- *What symptoms or signs improve*

- *How much those symptoms improve*

- *How fast they improve*

GET WELL NOW;
UNDERSTAND WHY
LATER

## CHAPTER 2:
## WHY CHOOSE PRESCRIPTFIT?

PrescriptFit® Medical Nutrition Therapy (MNT) offers a world of unique advantages over other approaches to weight loss and disease/symptom reduction. Primarily, MNT is focused on your health; weight loss is a side effect. It has been my experience that, for the most part, patients care much more about how they feel than a particular weight. In addition, they want to feel better immediately. PrescriptFit offers these solutions. Results are fast!

PrescriptFit is healthy, flexible, cost effective, and designed for long-term success. Now that we know WHAT PrescriptFit involves (covered in chapter 1), let's look at WHO it's designed for as well as HOW and WHY it is successful.

1. **WHO?** — PrescriptFit is designed for those suffering from some level of obesity and specific medical conditions, which improve no matter how overweight one is or how much they lose.

   PrescriptFit not only improves symptoms of various illnesses, it frequently results in being able to decrease medications (only if your healthcare provider recommends this approach), losing excess fat, and prolonging life. As you will learn in section C, medical experts recommend MNT as the first line of treatment for many medical conditions and medication add-on therapy for other conditions.

2. **HOW?** — When you are not feeling or functioning well, you want results now! The PrescriptFit Plan is designed to gain measurable improvement—fast! Follow the Plan precisely for best and fastest results.

# PRESCRIPTFIT
MEDICAL NUTRITION THERAPY ■ ■ ■ ■ ■ ■ ■

# ∽ CHAPTER 2: WHY CHOOSE PRESCRIPTFIT? ∽

3. **WHY?** — Feeling well is vital for long-term motivation. Staying well requires understanding why you felt better to begin with, so you can stick with the PrescriptFit Plan forever. Following the Plan is highly educational — it positively reinforces when disease or symptoms improve and negatively reinforces when symptoms return (due to abandoning the Plan or adding a new Food Phase that results in symptom return).

*Patients seek healthcare provider help when they no longer feel well — when they are sick! They are happy and motivated when they improve or get well. They are less likely to want to return to that poor state of health if the improvement is substantial and measurable.*

## THE HEALTHY SOLUTION

PrescriptFit involves daily medical treatment with amino acid-based supplements. As discussed in chapter 1, these amino acids are only now being discovered by the scientific community as having a "balancing" impact on the overproduction of cytokines that lead to a variety of illnesses. Using these natural amino acids rather than chemicals to balance metabolism and control hunger PLUS structured food groups that stress low-fat, low-calorie options, gives you a healthy controlled solution for today's dietary challenges.

Key components of PrescriptFit MNT (using the PrescriptFit products and MNT Food Phases) contribute to enhanced health and wellness by:

1. **Starting with PrescriptFit, a complete nutritional food** — One can have as much as they want and feel assured of their nutritional health (a multivitamin is mandatory; healthcare provider follow up on medication and symptoms is vital).

*Some may want to remain in Food Phase I for several months if under close supervision by their healthcare provider.*

2. **Helping fight disease using branched-chain amino acids** — Recent research links these to safely fighting inflammation, cardiac disease, metabolic disorders, and mental health problems.

## PRESCRIPTFIT
MEDICAL NUTRITION THERAPY ▪ ▪ ▪ ▪ ▪ ▪ ▪

©2017 Stanford A. Owen, MD

3. **Not eliminating any food groups** — MNT Food Phases focus on low-fat, low-calorie, structured food groups without eliminating or over-emphasizing any single food group.

4. **Letting you pinpoint where and how symptoms improve** — Measures of improvement are tracked using "clinically significant measures": lab tests your healthcare provider's office performs (e.g., blood pressure, blood sugar, cholesterol, etc.)

*For those with illness, medical supervision is mandatory.*

5. **Recommending collaboration with your healthcare provider** — Talk with your provider before beginning the Plan; share information from this book and discuss how to monitor symptom change as you progress through the Food Phases.

6. **Being inclusive** — Any and every family member can use and learn from the MNT Plan. The more you involve your family, friends, work colleagues, AND your healthcare provider, the more likely you will be to achieve optimum health.

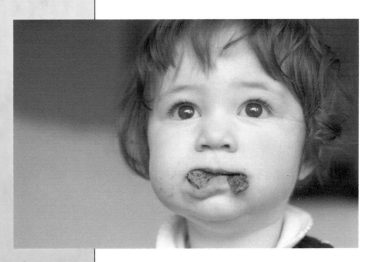

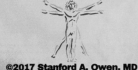

# ~ CHAPTER 2: WHY CHOOSE PRESCRIPTFIT? ~

## THE FLEXIBLE SOLUTION

Forget all the "rules" of diets you've tried in the past. MNT incorporates real-world approaches that give you the flexibility to make healthy eating and wellness a permanent lifestyle change. The PrescriptFit eating Plan lets you structure:

> **How and when you consume your "treatment" doses of PrescriptFit supplement** — Enjoy milk shakes, soups, and puddings before meals or instead of meals every day.

> **How long you follow each of the structured Food Phases** — Introduce new food groups one at a time for three-, seven-, or fourteen-day periods designed to target the level of risk you face from illness and the rate at which you want/ need to lose weight.

> **In what order you add Food Phases** — If you have allergies, are vegetarian, don't know how to cook, or just plain don't like a particular food group, you can skip or rearrange the order in which you add food groups. The important thing is to add one group at a time for the duration that fits your risk level/weight loss rate goal.

> **Eating out, at holiday gatherings, on vacation** — PrescriptFit's "splurging" concept allows eight splurge meals each month — enough to go on a cruise, spend a long weekend eating Mom's home cooking, or just maintain that Friday night pizza tradition your family adores.

> **How to improve results** — Start back at Phase 1 and try a longer duration or perhaps add more exercise or reduce the number of splurge meals per month. It's your diet, your solution.

*Limit foods in Phases 9-13 to "splurge" meals (see chapter 7).*

*This is the only diet strategy that recognizes that we all have to splurge from time to time. PrescriptFit gives you a simple way to manage and ENJOY those times.*

## PRESCRIPTFIT
MEDICAL NUTRITION THERAPY ▪ ▪ ▪ ▪ ▪ ▪ ▪

©2017 Stanford A. Owen, MD

# SECTION A: TAKING CONTROL...

*There are times in our lives when our kids, our parents, our jobs, or our friends all have a major impact on when, how, what, and where we eat.*

The "splurge" concept was born of the understanding that life is unpredictable. "Stuff" happens. Schedules go by the wayside. Partying occurs. Tragedy hits. Events occur in our lives every day that are more important than the next meal or recipe preparation. The ultimate flexibility — "falling off the wagon" — is NO BIG DEAL with PrescriptFit. When people have too many splurge meals or don't stick to the initial phases of the Plan, it's NO BIG DEAL. You just get back on the program and move on. PrescriptFit is a learning experience, not a "pass" or "fail" test. In fact, your body will tell you what to do. For most people, symptoms such as pain, inflammation, acid reflux, and others quickly return when they either fail to maintain amino acid supplement intake and/or indulge in too many high-calorie/high-fat meals. Relief comes quickly once you get back on the Plan.

Splurging is also incorporated with the PrescriptFit MNT plan based on "anticipation science." This is the science that is the anchor of the gaming industry (gambling). It seems all

## REAL-WORLD FLEXIBILITY

1. Don't avoid eating out. Once you've completed the first two or three Food Phases (based on how you choose to structure them), you will be able to go out to any restaurant and enjoy poultry, seafood, vegetables, salads, nuts, fruit, and eggs in any quantity you wish.

2. Having a busy week with lots of overtime at the office? PrescriptFit shakes, puddings, soups, and snack bars are an easy, "no-brainer" way to stay full, satisfied, and feeling great. Then, when the deadlines are over, enjoy that "splurge" meal you've not had time for. PrescriptFit is the flexible solution designed for your unique lifestyle.

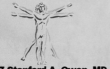

©2017 Stanford A. Owen, MD

**PRESCRIPTFIT**
MEDICAL NUTRITION THERAPY ■ ■ ■ ■ ■ ■ ■

# CHAPTER 2: WHY CHOOSE PRESCRIPTFIT?

mammals like to anticipate what's in the future and that most mammals will create anticipation for enjoyment. PrescriptFit Plan simply adds anticipation as a normal behavior. With a new food group just around the corner, anticipation is always in place.

*Anticipation may well be an ancient instinct that developed for unknown reasons. All we know is that it works.*

## Pick the Phase Duration that's Right for YOU

| Level of Risk/ Weight Loss Rate (estimated pounds/week depending on initial wt.) | Medical Health | Days/ Phase | Medical Attention Needed During MNT |
|---|---|---|---|
| Low/Slow (1-2) | • Not taking prescription medication for specific illness<br>• Conditions not yet life-threatening | 3 | |
| Medium/Moderate (2-3) | • Taking prescription medications for chronic illness<br>• Have significant symptoms<br>• Stable and not at risk for imminent death | 7 | • Need frequent monitoring of condition<br>• Should be managed by a physician during MNT |
| High/Rapid (3-6) | • Taking prescription medications for chronic illness<br>• Have symptoms that are disabling and require frequent physician exams<br>• At risk for death or serious disability | 14 | • Need frequent monitoring of condition<br>• MUST be managed by a physician during MNT |

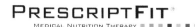

PRESCRIPTFIT
MEDICAL NUTRITION THERAPY

©2017 Stanford A. Owen, MD

# ~ Section A: Taking Control... ~

*If you use PrescriptFit shakes, soups, or puddings to replace one or two meals each day ($2-4/meal), you will save considerably over "normal" diets and fast food ($4-8/meal).*

*PrescriptFit is one of the best investments you can make in your health and your future. It pays back astonishing dividends!*

## THE COST-EFFECTIVE SOLUTION

All weight-loss diets cost money for special foods/supplements, "membership," and/or coaching. PrescriptFit involves a cost for purchasing the PrescriptFit supplement products; however, using these products is less expensive overall than following other commercial diet plans we've compared. Realize that some diets structure costs based on complete foods provided, others include fees for participation in the program, and others allow for purchasing your own food (at grocers or in restaurants) for some or all meals.

**What do we actually spend on the food we eat?** Based on U.S. Department of Agriculture and the Food Marketing Institute published data, the average family spends between $500 and $1,000 per month with food prepared at home, not including eating out. The USDA also estimates that over 40 percent of all meals are eaten out of the home in most urban settings, which might raise the family expenditure to about $1,300/month. Given these figures, PrescriptFit products are significantly less expensive than the average North American food bill (groceries plus dining out). Fast food or restaurant food is considerably more expensive.

### Data Sources:

- Food Marketing Institute. (2014). U.S. Grocery Shopper Trends

- Rao, M., Afshin, A. Singh, G., Mozaffarian, D. (December 2013). Do healthier foods and diet patterns cost more than less healthy options? A systematic review and meta-analysis. BMJ Open 2013;3:e004277 doi:10.1136.bmjopen-2013-00427

- U.S. Department of Agriculture Economic Research Service. (Nov. 17, 2014). Table 2— Food at home: Total expenditures; Table 10 — Food away from home as a share of food expenditures. http://www.ers.usda.gov/data-products/food-expenditures.aspx

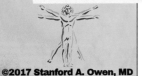

©2017 Stanford A. Owen, MD

## PRESCRIPTFIT
MEDICAL NUTRITION THERAPY ■ ■ ■ ■ ■ ■ ■

**But, won't adding all those "healthy" fresh foods to the PrescriptFit meals cost a lot more at the grocery store?** You are right that many foods — seafood, fresh fruits, and fresh vegetables — typically cost more than high-fat, high-calorie processed foods. In fact, according to a study published in December of 2013 by the Harvard School of Public Health (HSPH), the higher cost of healthier food choices is equal to about $10-$11 a week per person. Some of the cost involved food items just not being available in easily accessible stores; some cost reflected simply higher prices for the healthier item due to volume of product sold. What's the solution if you're on a limited budget? Consider your current spending each day for food, and try this experiment:

*EATING COSTS US MONEY, NO MATTER HOW YOU LOOK AT IT.*

1.  Replace one meal a day totally with a PrescriptFit shake, pudding, or soup.

2.  Have a PrescriptFit shake, pudding, or soup right before you eat a regular meal, which will reduce the amount you want to eat during that meal.

If you track what you actually spend with this approach, you may very well find that healthier eating isn't more expensive after all.

**But what about your overall budget?** How much do you currently spend on medications — both prescription and over the counter? How much do you spend out of pocket each year on medical office visits related to chronic illness? It is very likely that, because balancing cytokines with amino acid supplements reduces symptoms of many chronic illnesses, you will start to see significant savings in medical costs. No doubt about it — chronic illness is an expensive way to live!

*What would feeling better mean for your productivity at work and at home? What could that productivity mean in terms of career advancement? Although we may not be able to put a dollar figure to these considerations, we all know that when we feel good, everything just goes better.*

**PRESCRIPTFIT**
MEDICAL NUTRITION THERAPY ▪ ▪ ▪ ▪ ▪ ▪

# ~ SECTION A: TAKING CONTROL... ~

**PrescriptFit's unique nutrition treatment strategy is:**

- *Safe*
- *Medically credible*
- *Satisfying*
- *Easy*
- *Socially acceptable*
- *Instructive*
- *Intuitive*
- *Inexpensive*
- *Reproducible*
- *Measurable*

## THE LONG-TERM SOLUTION

PrescriptFit offers a unique approach to weight loss and wellness that helps people make permanent lifestyle changes vital for living longer, more productive lives. **How?** The PrescriptFit MNT Plan:

> **Avoids deprivation** — No foods are excluded permanently.

> **Lets you eat the size portions you want** — Using PrescriptFit supplement shakes, puddings, and soups as medical treatment before and/or instead of some meals lets you eat more of the allowable foods in the Phase you are currently in.

> **Gives you something "to look forward to"** — MNT lets you consistently add Food Phases, teaches you how to prepare foods in new ways that taste great, and allows eight "splurge" meals a month after completing Phase 8.

> **Keeps you from getting bored** — MNT holds your interest by focusing on measures, providing new methods of food preparation, and improving taste and variety.

Well-known weight-loss diets share a number of attributes, but studies of successful outcomes point to these five factors that appear to ensure long-term success: exercise, fruit and vegetable intake, accountability, record keeping, and supplement (shake) or special food product compliance. **Of these, the last item, supplement (shake) compliance, was the stronger predictor of success, statistically, than the other four factors combined.**

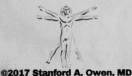

**PRESCRIPTFIT**
MEDICAL NUTRITION THERAPY ▪ ▪ ▪ ▪ ▪ ▪ ▪

# CHAPTER 3: HOW CAN YOU ENSURE SUCCESS?

Adequate preparation for permanently changing your diet, nutrition, and overall health is a big step. It requires several adjustments — in your attitude and perceptions, in your environment, in your day-to-day routines — that are critical to your long-term success. For many, dieting becomes a roller coaster of short-term change and long-term failure because they just weren't ready to make the changes the diet they chose required.

## GETTING YOUR HEAD IN THE GAME

**How we view what we eat or choose not to eat has a great deal to do with our attitudes and perceptions about food.** First of all, remember that the word, "diet," is not about how much you eat; it is about what foods you eat. What each person eats, when they eat, where they eat, and how they view these factors are very personal considerations. Improving our diet is all about balancing who we are, how we feel, and how we look with our eating habits.

It's important to realize that your general eating patterns and habits are greatly influenced by your upbringing. What time of day you choose to eat lunch or dinner, whether or not you eat snacks, whether or not you eat quietly or in big, family meals — all these factors are influenced by what you've grown up with. If mom's or grandma's special meals featured fried meats, lots of starches, and a bounty of yummy desserts, you probably keep those traditions sacred with your own families. Kids growing up in households where parents don't particularly like

*The experiences you've had to date with "dieting" have been different than those you will experience with the PrescriptFit MNT Plan.*

*The combination of amino acid supplements, structured food groups, and "legal" splurging gives you unprecedented ability to feel full and satisfied while eating less, not have to control portions in any Phase, be flexible in ways that fit your lifestyle and tastes, and never feel deprived.*

**These differences spell a whole new experience with diet.**

PRESCRIPTFIT
MEDICAL NUTRITION THERAPY ▪ ▪ ▪ ▪ ▪ ▪ ▪ ▪

©2017 Stanford A. Owen, MD

# ~ Section A: Taking Control... ~

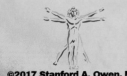

**Eating patterns, likes and dislikes, and family routines develop early and are very difficult to change.**

or prepare vegetables, fish, whole grains, and fruits will likely not fix those foods themselves when they become adults. There are also numerous emotional ties between love and food — approval for cleaning our plates, food as rewards for good behavior, comforting routines that include bedtime snacks.

Add to these challenges, the fact that our bodies change as we age, metabolizing the same foods differently. Also, the food industry has undergone tremendous changes, making a wealth of processed foods more available and less expensive over the past 50 years. All these packaged foods are heavily marketed and easily accessible to us every day. With our busy schedules, it's less likely that people will prepare and eat home-cooked, fresh foods on a regular basis.

Its no wonder so many people feel that they've failed to change their diets.

**Failure to control your weight is NOT a failure to avoid pleasure (greed) or to be disciplined (control of instinctual behavior), and it does not mean that you lack intelligence.** Failure to control weight is a complex issue that involves environmental, emotional, hormonal, instinctual, and motivational factors that cause more calories to enter your body than are being expended. Period.

**The solution:** Accept that failure is normal and must be confronted. Accept the challenges you've taken on and allow for the realities of your environment.

# ↝ CHAPTER 3: HOW TO ENSURE SUCCESS? ↜

Now let's focus on your goals; envisioning why you're doing battle with these lifestyle changes will help keep a positive perspective on the process. With PrescriptFit, you develop new discipline because you acquire new knowledge and skills, you have built-in accountability, AND you practice these new habits over time without fear of failure.Use the exercise below to help you hone in on your personal goals.

## EXERCISE 1: IDENTIFYING YOUR GOALS

### Why Am I Dieting?

**To feel better:**

__To help treat current medical problems
__To feel more energetic
__To reduce back/joint pain
__To enhance sports performance/increase stamina
__Other?

**To look better:**

__Be more attractive to a partner
__Be more accepted by family
__Be more accepted by friends
__Be more accepted at work
__Other?

### What are My Primary Goals?

Weight: _____
Shape (inches of waist, hips, etc.): _____

Posture: _____
Clothing sizes: _____
Prolonged life (to what age): _____
Financial viability (% of increased productivity): _____
Reduced medical costs (in $$$ or % of annual expenses): _____
Reduced disease symptoms: _____
Quality of life (physical, social, emotional): _____

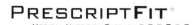

PRESCRIPTFIT
MEDICAL NUTRITION THERAPY ▪ ▪ ▪ ▪ ▪ ▪ ▪

©2017 Stanford A. Owen, MD

# ~ Section A: Taking Control... ~

## Learning About Food and Nutrition

Myths and misinformation about foods abound. These focus on high fat or low fat, food supplements or additives, artificial flavorings, or salt and sweeteners. Many people get sidetracked by these myths and avoid making changes in their diet or revert to familiar eating patterns out of fear or misinformation. The information below gives you the key points to remember about calories, proteins, carbohydrates, sweeteners, fats, and salt.

### Nutrition Basics

**Calories** — A calorie is a unit of heat liberated from food during digestion used for energy, growth, and repair.

**Proteins** — Proteins contain 4 calories/gram. When you eat protein in excess, it is converted either to carbohydrate for energy or to fat for storage. The "conversion" of protein to carbs or fat "uses up" 25 percent of calories in the protein molecule. Therefore, one can "cheat" on protein calories by 25 percent and not gain weight. Remember, that's just one-quarter more in your serving — not double the portions you usually have. In addition, protein does not stimulate the abnormal release of insulin and fat cell-produced cytokines, and therefore may not aggravate diabetes, pre-diabetes, hypertension, and lipids (cholesterol).

**Carbohydrates** — Carbohydrates contain 4 calories/gram and come from fruits and vegetables; breads, cereals, and other grains; milk and milk products, and sugar-sweetened foods (e.g., cakes, cookies, and beverages). Complex carbohydrates (from vegetables, fruits, whole grains, and beans) take longer to convert to glucose, giving our bodies time to effectively metabolize these foods without promoting the insulin resistance that leads to type 2 diabetes.

**Sweeteners** — Scientific research does NOT support the claims that artificial sweeteners can cause harm. In fact, the harmful effects of sugar far exceed those reported at times with saccharin or aspartame. Review the section on sweeteners on pages 36 through 40.

**Fats** — Fat contains 9 calories/gram. Unsaturated fat made from vegetable oil is less "toxic" to the cardiovascular system than saturated animal fat. Animal fat harms arteries and metabolism. Still, even unsaturated fats need to be consumed in moderation.

**Salt** — Salt is not harmful except in specific medical conditions, such as congestive heart failure (see section C). In fact, cytokines are much more likely than salt to cause fluid retention, which is why adding amino acids can be so effective in reducing fluid retention. Salt has no calories. Salt tastes great, especially when combined with other herbs and ingredients, making "new" foods taste more like what you're used to.

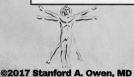

# CHAPTER 3: How to Ensure Success?

Some people simply refuse to learn new tastes, experiment with new flavors, methods of food preparation, or new buying habits because they just don't want to change. Change, by definition, is stressful.

**Skills are learned.** Most people learn eating habits, cooking skills, and nutrition "science" from parents or friends. Nutrition information in school is presented haphazardly and is often obsolete or single-minded. Nutrition classes rarely teach culinary or cooking skills. Each Food Phase of the PrescriptFit MNT Plan teaches skills you need for purchasing, preparing, and consuming foods that promote wellness.

*Skills develop with practice and can always be improved. Read, re-read, and practice the new skills presented with each Food Phase of the PrescriptFit MNT Plan.*

Medical nutrition, obesity, and food science researchers are in closer agreement about the kind of nutrition therapy used in PrescriptFit. There is an explosion of new information in every scientific journal. Some of this information is delivered by "sound bites" on the television or delivered out-of-context in newspapers, magazines, and via the Internet. We all "inhale" this scant new information as gospel, remember bits and pieces, and fix these bits as fact into our memories.

*Practice the skills you learned in previous Food Phases until you master them. Each time you use a recipe from a previous Food Phase, re-read that Food Phase.*

Each Food Phase of the PrescriptFit MNT Plan addresses that category of food with the latest science, nutrition, and calorie math. Each Phase provides best culinary methods for that food choice.

Learn.
Reinforce.
Practice.
Teach!

**The result** — accurate decision making when choosing food for yourself or family while quickly preparing more scrumptious meals.

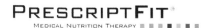

MANAGING FOOD FOR HEALTH JUST TAKES PRACTICE!

## PRESCRIPTFIT
MEDICAL NUTRITION THERAPY

## ~ SECTION A: TAKING CONTROL... ~

### UNDERSTANDING SWEETENERS

There is enormous misinformation among the public regarding natural and artificial sweeteners. Urban legend has ordained artificial sweeteners unsafe while science has ordained them among the safest food products ever studied. I doubt you will change your mind that the data proves them safe if you have developed a fixed conviction about artificial sweetener risk compared to the risks involved with ingesting sugar.

### THE PROBLEM WITH SUGAR

In my opinion, the most harmful substance in the human diet, in absolute number of people harmed, is sugar. Follow the path of the soda companies around the globe and track the obesity epidemic that has ensued to measure this impact. Ask the Chinese. Only 20 years ago, the average person in China worried more about starvation than overfeeding. Type 2 diabetes was rare. As a percentage of the population, China will soon have the greatest incidence of type 2 diabetes IN THE WORLD. What happened in China to produce this trend in only 20 years? A virus? No, it was soda companies and fast food companies bringing their fabulous tasty (and sugar-laden) foods to Mainland China.

> WHETHER THROWING A PARTY OR JUST PLANNING FOR DAILY SNACKING, REPLACING SUGAR SNACKS WITH FRUIT WILL CAUSE LESS RESISTANCE FROM KIDS AND SPOUSES.

Sugar causes harm in two ways. One is when mixed with liquids to form a drink. The other is when it is consumed along with fats.

**Sugar Mixed with Liquids** — Large amounts of sugar (20+ sugar packs/12 oz. drink) enter the blood stream very quickly, causing a spike

**PRESCRIPTFIT**
MEDICAL NUTRITION THERAPY ■ ■ ■ ■ ■ ■ ■

in the blood sugar concentration within minutes. Naturally occurring sugar, found in fruits and vegetables, is normally bound to the plant's fiber elements, which "hold" the sugar until acted upon by stomach acid or intestinal enzymes, slowing the release of sugar into the bloodstream.

The rate of sugar rise after a meal has been labeled the "glycemic index." Charts measuring glycemic indexes of different foods list liquid beverages as having the highest "glycemic index" of all food products. When someone with type 1 diabetes has a hypoglycemic attack from too much insulin, the classic treatment is gulping down a glass or two of orange juice as fast as possible.

Liquid sugar produces a sudden rise in insulin, a fall in an intestinal cytokine called GLP-1, then a myriad of downstream effects relating to other hormones that increase hunger while disturbing metabolism, producing:

> Elevated blood sugar
> Resistance to insulin
> Excessive fat formation
> Production of toxic protein cytokines, provoking inflammation in every organ

This cascade of metabolic changes caused by sugar is well documented in thousands of articles spanning decades.

**The Impact of Fructose** — We know the danger of sugar, especially fructose, which comes from fruits and vegetables and becomes harmful when ingested **without** the fiber from those fruits and vegetables and when ingested in large quantities. In my opinion, if fructose were introduced to the market today and had to gain FDA approval, it would fail, due to the overwhelming evidence of harm produced at the biochemical, cellular, and

*This impact of liquid sugar's glycemic index was best portrayed by Al Pacino in The Godfather. Toward the end of his life, the character suffers from diabetes: hands trembling, disoriented, sweaty, and off balance, which in the story is cured in 30 seconds by drinking orange juice!*

*Note: "Juiced" fruit has the sugar released from the fiber by the blender and is little different from juice obtained from the grocery.*

organ level. Essentially, fructose converts to fatty acids, the damaging form of cholesterol, and triglycerides — all of which our bodies store as fat in the liver and skeletal muscles. In addition, the way our livers process fructose results in lots of waste products and toxins, including uric acid, which elevates blood pressure and can cause gout.

In very small amounts, even pure sugar is relatively harmless (e.g., a cup of coffee with a pack of sugar or a sprinkle over berries). Harmless. It is the massive quantity in a rapid absorptive load that is dangerous.

**Sugar Mixed with Fat** — Sugar and refined carbohydrates are even more harmful when mixed with fat, especially saturated fat. This combination literally causes an explosion of toxic cytokine hormones from fat cells, intestines, liver, and brain. These sugar/fat combinations are familiar: cereal and milk, bread and butter, pasta and cream sauce, potatoes and sour cream, potatoes and grease (French fries), cookies, snacks, cakes, pies — the list is endless. Head to head, the sugar/fat combination is possibly more toxic than liquid sugar. Again, numerous studies in both animals and humans document this damage.

This combination of fat and sugar, in my opinion, IS the cause of type 2 diabetes, most hypertension, most sleep apnea, much joint pain and destruction, fatty liver, and a good portion of heart attack and stroke. Saturated fat and sugar are relegated to Phases 9-13 (starch introduced last) to avoid serious damage to metabolism until the patient has had a chance to heal, devoid of fat/carb toxins.

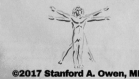

# CHAPTER 3: HOW TO ENSURE SUCCESS?

## SUGAR VS. ARTIFICIAL SWEETENERS

Artificial sweeteners, on the other hand, have been associated with zero deaths, no side effects (compared to placebo), and rare allergic or adverse events. More studies have been performed on artificial sweeteners, by more countries, than any compound in human history. No validated study has shown ill effect, even in massive doses larger than is possible for any human to consume in a lifetime. Many animal studies have been performed on many species with no ill effect. Aspartame, in particular, has been studied the most. If I had to defend myself in court about using aspartame vs. anything else I prescribe or recommend, I'd choose aspartame due to the overwhelming safety data.

In addition, due to the serious and prolonged attack on the Internet, aspartame and other sweeteners have been re-examined by U.S. government agencies at later dates, finding the same safety results. Former FDA Commissioner Arthur Hull Hayes stated, "Few compounds have withstood such detailed testing and repeated, close scrutiny, and the process through which aspartame has gone should provide the public with additional confidence of its safety." (Hayes, Federal Register, 1981)

Worldwide, the SCF (European FDA) in 2002 reaffirmed its safety support, and over 100 countries with scientific review panels for drug safety have approved aspartame use.

Still skeptical? Take a look at the web links, reports, and articles on the next page. Then, decide for yourself.

*Aspartame is one of the most widely consumed products in the world. Diet Coke® is now the #2-selling beverage in the world (behind Coca-Cola® Classic). With such massive consumption, ill effect would have long ago surfaced.*

**PRESCRIPTFIT**
MEDICAL NUTRITION THERAPY ▪ ▪ ▪ ▪ ▪ ▪ ▪

©2017 Stanford A. Owen, MD

REFERENCE LINKS FOR THOSE STILL SKEPTICAL
ABOUT ASPARTAME

1. American Cancer Society, www.cancer.org/aspartame

2. Centers for Disease Control. 1984. Evaluation of consumer complaints related to aspartame use. CDC, Atlanta, GA

3. European Commission. 1997. Scientific Committee on Food: Minutes of the 107th meeting of the Scientific Committee on Food. Pp. 9-10. June 12-13.

4. European Food Safety Authorisy. 2006. Opinion of the Scientific Panel AFC related to a new long-term carcinogenicity study on aspartame, May 5.

5. Food and Drug Administration, www.fda.gov/aspartame

6. Food and Drug Administration (FDA). 1981. Aspartame: Comissioner's final decision. *Fed Regist*. 46:38285-38308.

7. Food and Drug Administration (FDA) 1996b. FDA statement on aspartame, FDA Talk Paper, November 8.

8. National Cancer Institute, www.cancer.gov/aspartame

9. National Cancer Institute Cancer Facts. Artificial Sweeteners. http://cis.nci.nih.gov/fact/pdfdraft/3_risk/fs3 (2005)

10. National Toxicology Program. NTP Report on the Toxicology Studies of Aspartame in Genetically Modified Mice. 2005.

11. United Kingdom Committee on Carcinogenicity of Chemicals in Food, Consumer Products and the Environment, 14 July, 2005

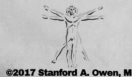

PRESCRIPTFIT
MEDICAL NUTRITION THERAPY ■ ■ ■ ■ ■ ■ ■

# CHAPTER 3: HOW TO ENSURE SUCCESS?

## BECOMING ACCOUNTABLE = BEST RESULTS

PrescriptFit provides built-in accountability to help you succeed with weight loss and symptom reduction. Accountability factors include:

*We all perform better when we're held accountable for our actions.*

> **Recording your progress on your PrescriptFit calendar** — Do it religiously. Don't lie or fudge. Learn from your efforts.

> **Relying on meal replacement use** — The more PrescriptFit shakes, soups, or puddings you use, the more you will lose and the better disease improvement you will experience. Studies show meal replacement use is the #1 predictor of diet success in our modern world.

> **Getting regular exercise** — Daily Over Duration! Do some exercise every day. Daily exercise of short duration will produce superior weight loss and medical benefit than the same total exercise done two or three times per week.

> **Involving others** — Connect with your healthcare provider, sponsor (who you buy PrescriptFit products from), or friend/coach. Have an important person review and accept your written results (on the calendar and questionnaires) and review your progress with you.

## Results = Knowledge X Skill X Accountability X Practice Over Time

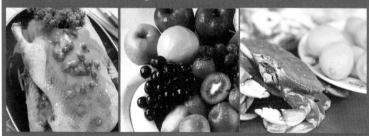

**PRESCRIPTFIT**
MEDICAL NUTRITION THERAPY ▪ ▪ ▪ ▪ ▪ ▪ ▪

When you start on PrescriptFit MNT, you will probably want to order the start-up kit that contains:

> The PrescriptFit Calendar — An invaluable tool for long-term success

> A three- to four-week supply (depending on use) of PrescriptFit products — the Vanilla Shake/Pudding Mix (regular or lactose-free formula), Chocolate Shake/Pudding Mix (regular or lactose-free formula), Beef Soup Mix, and Chicken Soup Mix.

> A sample assortment of delicious, calorie-free flavorings

### THE PRESCRIPTFIT CALENDAR

The Calendar provides space for you to record key factors related to the Plan each day, including:

> What Phase of the diet you are currently in

> The number of doses (scoops) of amino acids you consumed in PrescriptFit shakes/puddings/soups

> Time you spent exercising

> If you used a splurge meal (Phases 9–13)

Keeping consistent, accurate records of how you progress on the Plan will help you pinpoint what causes improvements or relapses you experience.

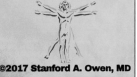

PRESCRIPTFIT®
MEDICAL NUTRITION THERAPY ▪ ▪ ▪ ▪ ▪ ▪ ▪

# CHAPTER 3: HOW TO ENSURE SUCCESS?

Other pages of the Calendar provide:

> A place to record baseline information

> Symptom Score Sheets to record your results every four weeks or after each phase

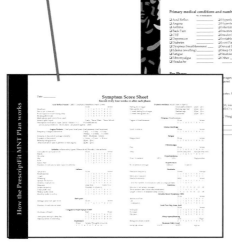

## PRESCRIPTFIT PRODUCTS

The PrescriptFit products are nutritionally complete supplements that come in vanilla or chocolate (lactose-free formulas available) for shakes and puddings as well as both a chicken and a beef soup mix. All mix with water (and crushed ice in the case of shakes) and are exceptionally flavorful without additional enhancement. All PrescriptFit products are formulated using egg whites and nonfat milk solids, and are fortified with additional branched-chain and essential amino acids: leucine, isoleucine, valine, lysine, histidine, and methionine in proprietary doses.

When using the Vanilla shake/pudding mix, take your favorite glass, fill 1/2 with water and 1/2 with ice; pour into blender with 2 scoops of Vanilla.

*"Essential" means the body cannot manufacture these amino acids from other dietary proteins.*

## PRESCRIPTFIT
MEDICAL NUTRITION THERAPY

©2017 Stanford A. Owen, MD

# SECTION A: TAKING CONTROL...

Blend until creamy. Add another scoop for an "ice cream" like effect. This product is delicious as creamer for coffee, when mixed with diet soft drinks, as a topping for your favorite fruit, or with nuts (Phase 5). The Chocolate shake/pudding mix is made from the finest imported cocoa and can be mixed the same as the Vanilla for optimum texture and flavor.

The lactose-free varieties of Vanilla and especially the Chocolate are very rich tasting. Use the Chocolate alone for maximal "chocoholic" satisfaction or mix with one scoop of Vanilla for a milky chocolate delight. Lactose free is the preferred product for those with irritable bowel syndrome (IBS).

The soup mixes include the same nutritionally complete formulas and are also fortified with branched-chain essential amino acids. The Chicken Soup is great as a hot drink or can be used as a thick sauce for meat or vegetable dishes. Beef soup gives a full-bodied beef taste that is especially good with meals or as a hot drink. Mix a scoop of each together for a real treat. Add vegetables, seafood, or poultry to the soup mix when you get to those Phases.

Other products in the PrescriptFit line include a variety of snack bars and crisps. Visit www.drdiet.com for more information.

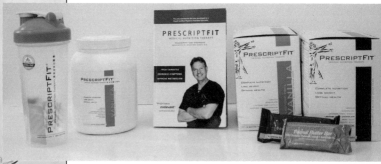

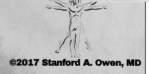

©2017 Stanford A. Owen, MD

**PRESCRIPTFIT**®
MEDICAL NUTRITION THERAPY

## CHAPTER 3: HOW TO ENSURE SUCCESS?

### FLAVORINGS

PrescriptFit flavorings are sugar-free, fat-free ways to bring fun variety to your shakes and puddings. Highly concentrated, these flavors encompass almost any taste — fruit, citrus, caramels and butter pecan, cheesecake, mint chocolate, cake batter, mocha — you name it. Use these flavorings to experiment with new toppings for fruits, blender drinks (if adding alcohol, don't try this until Phase 11), and varied milk shakes and puddings. Visit www.drdiet.com for more information.

### DOING ENVIRONMENTAL "CLEANUP"

For a few weeks before you begin the PrescriptFit MNT Plan, it's a good idea to do what we call the "Environmental Cleanup." This involves five crucial steps:

1. **Replace tempting foods not part of Phases 1-8 with the foods allowed during these Phases.** Success is more likely if tempting foods are not in the immediate environment — your home, workplace, and automobile. Alcoholics and cocaine addicts know relapse to drug use is more likely if they frequent situations where alcohol or cocaine is present. Food today tastes better than ever, is inexpensive, and is everywhere. No wonder many patients tell me they are food addicted and feel like they have no place to hide.

2. **Continue your usual diet pattern for four weeks BUT add in three doses** of PrescriptFit shakes, soups, or pudding mix in a single serving BEFORE (or instead of) breakfast and three doses **in a single shake, soup or pudding serving**

---

**Blender Tips:**

*Most blenders sold for non-commercial use are not designed for multiple use per day, especially when blending liquids with ice. To avoid burning out the motor of your home blender, be sure to use only crushed ice and to never use more ice than water in shake preparation.*

*Should you experience problems with blenders, consider purchasing a commercial bar blender (designed for daily, high-intensity use) from a restaurant supply company, or find a blender that is at least 25 years old at a garage sale or used appliance store. Apparently, they don't make 'em as good as they used to.*

*Be sure to remove ALL sugared drinks from your environment, including soda, juice, milk, and sports drinks. They are truly "empty" calories. Diet soda, sugar-free ice tea, and coffee with artificial sweetener and fat-free, non-dairy creamer are allowed during any Phase of the PrescriptFit MNT Plan.*

## PRESCRIPTFIT
MEDICAL NUTRITION THERAPY ▪ ▪ ▪ ▪ ▪ ▪ ▪ ▪

# ~ Section A: Taking Control... ~

**BEFORE (or instead of) dinner.** Why? The tactic will help you get accustomed to mixing tasty shakes, soups, and puddings and using them like "medication." Note any symptom improvement and/or weight loss.

3. **Do not change your exercise habits** (or lack thereof), but be sure and note what those habits are each day along with your weight. When you make a change in your exercise habits, you will want to compare results with this baseline condition.

4. **Measure your pre-Plan symptoms on the first Symptom Score Sheet located in the back of the Calendar.** You will use the second Symptom Score Sheet (and copies of it) to record symptoms and evaluate change after four weeks on the PrescriptFit MNT Plan (and at four-week intervals thereafter).

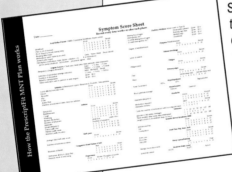

5. **Collaborate with your healthcare provider to ensure that your experience with** PrescriptFit MNT **is healthy** and successful (see the next section). Get medical advice on which Plan (14-day, 7-day, or 3-day per Phase) to choose for the health and weight loss goals you determined in Exercise 2 on page 48.

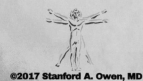

**PRESCRIPTFIT**
MEDICAL NUTRITION THERAPY ▪ ▪ ▪ ▪ ▪ ▪ ▪

# ☞ CHAPTER 3: HOW TO ENSURE SUCCESS? ☜

## TALKING TO YOUR HEALTHCARE PROVIDER ABOUT MNT

Most physicians receive very limited training on treating disease with diet. Medical schools don't emphasize nutrition or medical nutrition therapy as part of their regular curriculum. Once in practice, physicians learn from popular diet books or from professional publications, which contain bits and pieces of nutrition-related material.

When asked for diet advice, most healthcare providers refer to local dieticians or recommend a popular book. Some refer to commercial diet programs such as Weight Watchers. Ask. Share your Calendar and this book with your healthcare provider and ask his/her opinion. Show him/her the Healthcare Provider FAQs and the journal articles in appendix D. Have them contact us with questions at 888-460-6286.

Be sure to follow these guidelines:

> **Make an appointment with your healthcare provider BEFORE beginning the PrescriptFit MNT Plan.** Take this book and your Calendar, discuss the Plan, and review your current state of health including any baseline measures (blood pressure, weight, waist measurement, fasting blood sugar, cholesterol, triglycerides, etc.) that you will want to track as you proceed with the Plan. Use Exercise 2: Talking with Your Healthcare Provider on the next page to plan for covering important items during this initial visit. Many of the questions reflect current health guidelines. Write down your healthcare provider's answers to each question.

*Medical professional organizations recommend diet treatment of disease as the initial primary treatment for a number of medical conditions. Conditions or symptoms listed in the PrescriptFit materials reflect these professional guidelines as well as extensive publication, outcomes data, and/or experience.*

*The important thing is to embark on the PrescriptFit MNT Plan WITH your healthcare provider. You are not just trying to lose weight; you are actively pursuing health and reducing or eliminating symptoms of chronic illness. How your body reacts and what impacts that reaction might have on prescription medications you're taking demands close collaboration with your provider.*

**PRESCRIPTFIT**
MEDICAL NUTRITION THERAPY ■ ■ ■ ■ ■ ■ ■

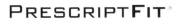

©2017 Stanford A. Owen, MD

# ~ SECTION A: TAKING CONTROL... ~

> **Use the Symptom/Disease Questionnaire** score sheets (in your Calendar and section C of this book) that you and your healthcare provider agree best reflect the measures you should follow. Most score sheets require you to reevaluate symptoms after Phase 1 and after every four weeks. Refer to the individual score sheets for more detail.

*If you choose the high-risk (rapid weight loss) approach, talk with your healthcare provider about more frequent contact.*

> **Make a follow-up appointment** four weeks past the time you begin PrescriptFit MNT. Review the results you've recorded on your Symptom/Disease Questionnaire score sheets with your healthcare

---

### EXERCISE 2: TALKING WITH YOUR HEALTHCARE PROVIDER

**Instructions: Check off those questions you want to ask your healthcare provider at your next appointment. Take along a note pad to record his/her answers.**

❑ What is your experience with medical nutrition therapy?

❑ What diet recommendations do you currently make? To whom do you refer patients for nutritional counseling?

❑ What impacts might MNT have on me personally given my health and current medications?

❑ What baseline measures on the Disease/Symptom Questionnaires can be monitored over time for improvement?

❑ Are there other measures I should monitor?

❑ What is my body mass index (BMI), and is this a problem for me?

❑ What is my waist circumference and does it possibly signal insulin resistance problems?

❑ Are my triglycerides over 150 mg/dL?

❑ Is my HDL cholesterol less that 40 (men) or 50 (women) mg/dL?

❑ Is my blood pressure greater than 130/85 mm Hg?

❑ Is my fasting glucose greater than 110 mg/dL?

❑ Should MNT be a first-line treatment for my problems? Or, add-on treatment?

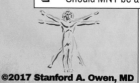

**PRESCRIPTFIT**®
MEDICAL NUTRITION THERAPY ■ ■ ■ ■ ■ ■ ■

provider to evaluate what impact the changes you've made are having on your symptoms.

> **DO NOT discontinue or alter the way you take any prescription medications,** even if your symptoms disappear. Always contact your healthcare provider before making any changes to medications.

## OVERCOMING OBSTACLES

Know the obstacles to improved health from the "get-go." The greatest obstacle to most is the food environment provided by loved ones: spouses, children, parents, and friends. We are literally "loved" to death with food in modern culture. Parents would never think of offering their drug-addicted teen more addictive drug, yet those same parents allow their socially shunned, obese child to consume foods likely to cause obesity.

In my experience, most patients feel their own medical problems are not the concerns of others. "It's my problem, not yours," and "You should not have to suffer for me," are typical "martyr" statements. Likewise, many patient family members feel exactly the same —"It's your problem, not mine." In reality, everyone pays for chronic disease and misery related to obesity via the monthly health insurance bill as well as physical, mental, or social disability.

PrescriptFit allows every major category of food. The only food group that you should completely avoid is sugared beverages (soft drinks, juices, sport drinks, and milk). There are NO redeeming features to anyone consuming these "empty calories." Avoiding these caloric beverages should be a family affair.

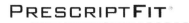

PRESCRIPTFIT
MEDICAL NUTRITION THERAPY ■ ■ ■ ■ ■ ■ ■

©2017 Stanford A. Owen, MD

# ~ Section A: Taking Control... ~

**Willpower Just Doesn't Work**

Family members are often more reluctant to remove bread, snacks, crackers, cakes, pies, and pasta compared to caloric beverages from the household. Alternatives (fruit, vegetables, and PrescriptFit snack bars) should be discussed and negotiation must occur. You will need to communicate to family members that "willpower" cannot overcome tempting delights. It is relatively easy to say "no" to bringing a pie into the house. It is impossible not to eat the pie once in the house.

### PLANNING FOOD/PRODUCT PREPARATION

Section B includes tips for shopping, buying, seasoning, and preparing foods within different Phases that you will want to review.

*Use the "shopping lists" provided for Phases 1-8 recipes to get started creating the pantry items you need to make the Plan a success.*

Revisit the organization of your kitchen. Perhaps you have a cabinet or other space you can devote completely to your PrescriptFit product prep. Gather together your blender, measuring cups/spoons, PrescriptFit shake and soup mixes, flavorings, and condiments (such as fat-free, sugar-free gelatin desserts and puddings and other seasonings) in a single location to make it easy to quickly prepare your PrescriptFit doses. No one wants to take the time to pull out and replace all these components if scattered about the kitchen.

Don't let yourself run out of essentials. There are too many high-fat, high-sugar alternatives just around the corner that take less time to pick up than going to the grocery store. Be sure to stock up each week on what you need for the Food Phases you're currently working with.

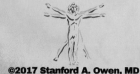

**PRESCRIPTFIT**®
MEDICAL NUTRITION THERAPY ■ ■ ■ ■ ■ ■ ■

# ~ CHAPTER 3: HOW TO ENSURE SUCCESS? ~

## PLANNING FOR EXERCISE

Exercise recommended for the PrescriptFit MNT Plan is very simple. After years of treating patients, both successfully and unsuccessfully, I've learned that exercise is a major predictor of weight loss success. As you would expect, those who do the most exercise most consistently lose the most weight, improve the most medically, and decrease the most their need to take medications.

What might seem somewhat paradoxical is that the amount of exercise is not as important as the consistency of exercise. Those who do any amount exercise every day will generally have better outcomes than those who exercise a few times per week, even if that exercise is considerably more intense and more prolonged.

Modest walking produces health benefits nearly as great as with intense exercise. The key words are "health benefits." Having a "buffed" and lean body may take large amounts of daily exercise, but health improvement can be registered with much less effort.

PrescriptFit MNT suggests doing 15 minutes of exercise per day, preferably broken into two or three separate sessions of five to 10 minutes each for greatest benefit.

### Why would such meager activity bring health results?

1. **"Daily" is a key theme in exercise.** Daily performance of any health habit shapes the day with compliance of other health habits, like compliance with diet.

2. **Five to 10 minutes will never interrupt other activities**; thus, the excuse that "I just don't have time" tends to go away.

*Muscle manufactures and alters cytokine production. Daily muscle use affects daily cytokine metabolism.*

*Learning to use exercise time most productively is important. Exercise devices can be helpful for those in hot, cold, or rainy environments. They are inexpensive. Buy them and use them every day!*

PRESCRIPTFIT
MEDICAL NUTRITION THERAPY ■ ■ ■ ■ ■ ■ ■

©2017 Stanford A. Owen, MD

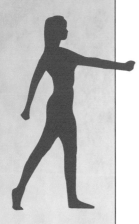

## SECTION A: TAKING CONTROL...

3. **Fifteen minutes is equivalent to walking one mile.** One mile is a measurable number and is the "payback" number (100 calories burned) we use to emphasize calorie value in food. Is one glass of juice or a bowl of cereal once per day worth 1.5 miles (150 calories) of walking payback per day? I doubt it!

4. **Fifteen minutes adds up to total fat loss.** One mile of walking per day (15 minutes) burns 100 calories in a 150-pound person. That adds up to 2,800 calories per month.

   One pound of fat contains 3,500 calories. Therefore, the 150-pound person would burn up about 8 pounds per year (and the 300-pound person 16 pounds per year) with 15 minutes of exercise per day. In five years, 40 pounds would be lost.

   If the 15 minutes are used to improve postural strength, such as abdominal strengthening exercises, you will realize additional benefit for painful and damaged back and joint structures.

*Be sure to record your time spent exercising each day on your PrescriptFit Calendar.*

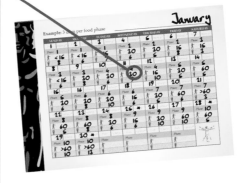

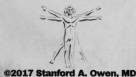

**PRESCRIPTFIT**®
MEDICAL NUTRITION THERAPY ■ ■ ■ ■ ■ ■ ■

# CHAPTER 3: HOW TO ENSURE SUCCESS?

## WORKING WITHIN YOUR LIFESTYLE

Okay, so you might wonder how to make PrescriptFit work for you if you travel extensively for business, work in a location where food preparation isn't really possible, or just don't know anything about cooking.

The built-in flexibility of the PrescriptFit MNT Plan is designed for success no matter what life throws at you. In any case, you will probably need to start Phase I of the Plan when you can be at home for the first couple of days at least. This will let you prepare the shakes/puddings as often as necessary using a blender and crushed ice and adding allowable flavors from your pantry. Of course, this will be more of a challenge if you select the 7-day or 14-day Plans; however, once you go off to work, the Soup mixes can be mixed in a cup with water and heated in the microwave for lunch. You can make a shake or two ahead and freeze, letting it thaw to the right consistency by mid morning.

One of the best ways to overcome dislike of cooking is to take one day a week and find a friend to cook with. Make larger quantities of soups, fruit salads, and baked/grilled dishes that you can "warm up" after work during the week. Enjoy the time together and learn from one another. You can also do this with your own family, creating some new quality time that promotes mutual understanding about foods and healthy eating patterns.

If you tend to eat out fairly often, use some of the strategies in the "Tips for Business Travelers" (on the previous page) to make dining out work for you.

*By following the cooking instructions in each of the Food Phases in Section B and trying the recipes at www.drdiet. com, you can learn just a few skills to make following the PrescriptFit MNT Plan a success.*

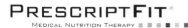

**PRESCRIPTFIT**
MEDICAL NUTRITION THERAPY

©2017 Stanford A. Owen, MD

# ~ Section A: Taking Control... ~

Because you can choose the number of days per Phase, the order in which you add Phases 2-8, and when to plan your "splurge" meals once you hit Phase 9, you have a great deal of flexibility for any lifestyle challenges you currently face. Remember, the PrescriptFit MNT Plan is designed to be YOUR Solution!

## TIPS FOR THE BUSINESS TRAVELER

- Create a small bag with individual servings of PrescriptFit product and small flavoring bottles to take with you on the road.

- Consider purchasing a MagicBullet™ blender (sold in various retail stores and over the Internet at www.buythebullet.com). It is small, lightweight, and very powerful.

- Once you've hit Phase 2 and beyond, scope out restaurants in the areas you travel (online or from feedback from business colleagues in that location) that cater to those on low-fat, low-calorie diets. For example, some restaurant chains feature entrees with specific calorie, fat, and Weight Watcher point totals. Call ahead and ask about grilled fish or chicken entrees as well as steamed vegetable plates; when you arrive, be sure to request your meals without sauces but with lemon wedges or salsa or Tabasco sauce.

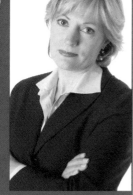

- Almost every town has a grocery store with a salad bar; try getting a salad WITHOUT cheese and high-calorie/high-fat dressing to go and picnicking in a nearby park.

- If your travel budget allows, ask to stay in "suites" hotels that feature in-room microwaves and refrigerators; stock up on fruit, shrimp cocktail, or microwavable grilled chicken wings to have in the room (depending on the Phase you're in).

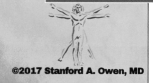

**PRESCRIPTFIT®**
MEDICAL NUTRITION THERAPY ▪ ▪ ▪ ▪ ▪ ▪ ▪

# NOTES

**QUESTIONS?**

EMAIL DR. OWEN AT
DROWENMD@DRDIET.COM

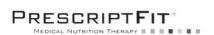

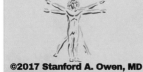

PRESCRIPTFIT®
MEDICAL NUTRITION THERAPY

# NOTES

QUESTIONS?

EMAIL DR. OWEN AT
DROWENMD@DRDIET.COM

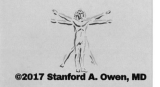

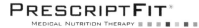

PRESCRIPT**FIT**

MEDICAL NUTRITION THERAPY

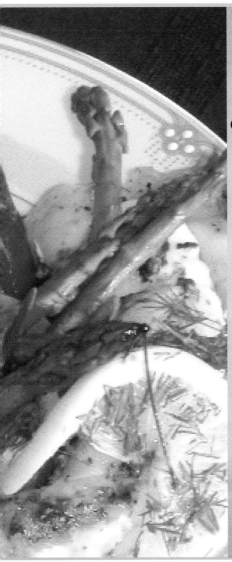

# DIVING IN – THE STRUCTURED FOOD PHASE APPROACH

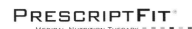
PRESCRIPTFIT®
MEDICAL NUTRITION THERAPY

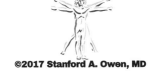

# TABLE OF CONTENTS

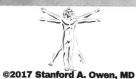

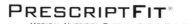

PRESCRIPTFIT®
MEDICAL NUTRITION THERAPY

# Section B: Diving In –
# The Structured Food Phase Approach

## Chapter 4: Overview of the Food Phase Strategy

Think of the PrescriptFit® Medical Nutrition Therapy (MNT) Food Phase Strategy as a personal training regimen, in which you work with YOU – your own personal trainer – one step at a time, building new skills and experience until you have achieved your desired level of fitness. What could be easier and more personal than having yourself and your own body as your trainers!

You will start at the beginning with the first food phase and gradually add food groups in each subsequent phase until your food plan includes all major food groups. You will not be deprived of any food. Each time you transition to a new food group, your body will communicate with you, the trainer, about its experience. Your body will tell you which foods make you feel more or less energetic, which relieve or exacerbate symptoms, and which cause you to lose or add weight. Just as a personal trainer adjusts exercise strategies for an athlete, you will be able to adjust your food plan for optimum health.

PrescriptFit MNT puts you in charge. You can design your own eating styles to fit any taste, budget, or cultural preferences. "But I hate seafood," you're thinking. Or, "I love dairy products." If you want to gain control of your health, you need an open mind about the variety of foods available. On the other hand, if you have food allergies, or if you have chosen a vegetarian lifestyle, this book will suggest ways to modify your eating plan to accommodate those needs.

*PrescriptFit MNT stresses:*

- *A Food Phase Strategy that allows you to isolate those foods that most impact how you feel*

- *PrescriptFit supplements that both taste great and dramatically reduce a number of illness symptoms*

- *Flexibility to spend 3, 7, or 14 days in each Food Phase, depending on the intensity of your disease symptoms and your personal preferences*

- *A healing and education period that lets you learn to adjust your buying, seasoning, and cooking habits for optimum health*

- *An oh-so-needed splurge element that gives you opportunities every week to eat socially and to treat yourself to the things you love*

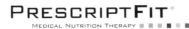

PRESCRIPTFIT®
MEDICAL NUTRITION THERAPY ▪ ▪ ▪ ▪ ▪ ▪ ▪

©2017 Stanford A. Owen, MD

# SECTION B: DIVING IN...

Each Food Phase is designed to teach you a fundamental principle: How your body reacts to different food groups. By experiencing each Phase in a prescribed sequence, you'll learn what your body needs.

As you begin each Phase, you'll be reminded of the diet components that you will use consistently throughout the Plan and beyond as you maintain your weight. And, you'll be reminded to use your PrescriptFit Calendar to record your splurge meals each week.

| | MNT GOAL | FOOD OPTIONS | YOUR OBJECTIVES |
|---|---|---|---|
| **Phase 1** | Medical Treatment | PrescriptFit Supplements (Shakes, Soups, Puddings) | • Conditioning for your new eating regimen<br>• Eliminating toxic cytokines |
| **Phases 2 – 8** | Healing & Education | Phase 2: Seafood<br>Phase 3: Poultry<br>Phase 4: Vegetables<br>Phase 5: Eggs<br>Phase 6: Nuts<br>Phase 7: Fruit<br>Phase 8: Snacks<br><br>PrescriptFit Shakes, Soups, and Puddings | • Learning food science, nutrition, and culinary techniques — one phase at a time<br>• Continuing to eliminate toxic cytokines |
| **Phases 9 – 13** | Splurging | Phases 2-8<br>Phases 9-13 (as two splurge meals/week)<br><br>PrescriptFit Shakes, Soups, and Puddings | • Gradually adding higher-fat/ higher-calorie components of a complete lifestyle<br>• Learning which food groups cause harm<br>• Continuing to eliminate toxic cytokines |

PRESCRIPTFIT®
MEDICAL NUTRITION THERAPY ▪ ▪ ▪ ▪ ▪ ▪ ▪

# ☞ Chapter 4: Strategy Overview ☜

## PRESCRIPTFIT FOOD PHASE STRATEGY — CORE PRINCIPLES

Strategy is everything when predicting success with any diet intervention. Layers of strategy are incorporated into the PrescriptFit MNT Food Phases. It is not important to understand why the "Phase" strategy was developed to be successful but it will help you respond to those who might try to derail you from succeeding. It's also not important why and it would take volumes to cover the psychology involved with group diet behavior. Those of you who have attempted serious dietary change know what I mean.

The core principles underlying PrescriptFit Food Phase strategy include:

> Safety
> Effectiveness
> Anticipation
> Discovery
> Surprise
> Reinforcement
> Education
> Group Cohesion (fitting in)
> Discipline
> Choice/Autonomy

## SAFETY

**All treatment of any medical condition should be both safe and effective.** Agreed-upon standards should be met. While unique in approach, PrescriptFit complies with dietary science; then it adds the extensive 30-year experience from daily patient care of those suffering from serious nutrition-related disease.

**Engineered Food** — PrescriptFit strategy uses an engineered food product alone as the initial treatment. It is comprised of egg white, calcium casienate, and micronized amino acids. The

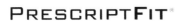

# SECTION B: DIVING IN...

balance of macronutrients is approximately 50 percent protein, 50 percent complex carbohydrate, and zero fat. Each dose (scoop) contains 100 calories and 10 grams of high-quality protein (plus amino acids). Minimal protein requirements to prevent muscle breakdown (while dieting) are met if five (5) doses of PrescriptFit are consumed daily (50 grams). The 50 percent carbohydrate is used for cell energy, allowing the proteins to be used for growth and repair of cells. Micronized amino acids (e.g., leucine and isoleucine, valine, lysine, histidine, methionine in proprietary doses) provide insulin-resistant cells a mechanism for getting nutrition for both energy and repair. Once repaired, cells are then able to again utilize insulin properly, and insulin resistance improves or resolves completely.

It is impossible to achieve minimal nutrition protein requirements with less than 50 grams of protein per day (five doses of PrescriptFit). **One should never consume less than 50 grams of protein and 500 calories per day for any length of time, as it can cause muscle breakdown (including heart muscle breakdown).**

**Very Low Calorie Diet** — A diet above 500 calories per day up to 800 calories per day requires a pre-measured engineered food to meet standards for safe nutrition. "Natural " food cannot be safely consumed at doses this low. A diet in this range is defined as a Very Low Calorie Diet (VLCD). VLCD diets, including PrescriptFit when used alone, have been proven extremely safe and effective at improving disease and metabolism. More than 30 years' experience and numerous publications have proven the safety of VLCDs by researchers and commercial nutrition companies.

Diets in the VLCD calorie range need to be medically monitored. This is especially true

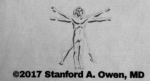

PRESCRIPTFIT®
MEDICAL NUTRITION THERAPY ▪ ▪ ▪ ▪ ▪ ▪ ▪

# CHAPTER 4: STRATEGY OVERVIEW

if you are on medications that may require adjustment (usually lower dose or discontinuance). Medications may need to be down regulated within the first week of starting a VLCD. Patients using insulin, gliburide, or glimiperide should be especially alert for hypoglycemia. Diabetes, hypertension, heart disease, and lipid disorders often require lower doses of medication or even discontinuance. Metabolism improvement is measured in hours or days, so vigilance early in the process is imperative.

Because patients often feel so much better, discontinue medications, and lose large amounts of weight quickly, many wish to remain on the VLCD much longer than 3, 7, or 14 days. This is perfectly safe as long as monitored by a healthcare provider. Many patients chose to remain in Phase 1 (shakes, soups, puddings) for months.

## EFFECTIVENESS

**Any diet strategy chosen should be effective for the desired goals, which can be achieved if compliance is high.** Therefore, compliance and effectiveness are linked, as evidenced by countless published scientific articles (and common sense).

PrescriptFit Phases were designed to achieve compliance by:

> Starting with foods less likely to cause diseased metabolism (Phase 1-8 foods)

> Managing, *not excluding,* those foods likely to cause harm (Phase 9-13 foods).

The PrescriptFit strategies were chosen because they are effective, even if custom design causes a deviation from the usual recommended Phases. The foods were chosen in order of most likely for

*Of patients using PrescriptFit products alone, the patient who had the longest stretch on VLCD was a five-year-old who remained on the products for 18 months. He lost 120 pounds and took his first-ever steps walking, which had previously been prohibited by his near-fatal weight. Eight years later, this teenager is still using PrescriptFit products as the primary food in his arsenal to stay alive and healthy.*

*Throughout this section, you will find brief stories of people with different lifestyles who have found their own ways to successfully adapt the Plan to their particular realities of work, home, family life, and travel.*

## PRESCRIPTFIT®
MEDICAL NUTRITION THERAPY ▪ ▪ ▪ ▪ ▪ ▪ ▪

©2017 Stanford A. Owen, MD

# Section B: Diving In...

even diehard healthy food "rebels." Compliance is complicated but involves taste, satiety, convenience, familiarity, cost, and inclusiveness. Effectiveness involves both biochemical effectiveness and behavioral effectiveness. PrescriptFit achieves both.

Improvement may differ by medical condition and patient as well as by social situation. Effectiveness of one process (diabetes) may be slightly different than for other processes (hypertension, lipid disorders, fatty liver). Most patients' diabetes is controlled in days or weeks, while the occasional patient may require weeks or months to gain control. Effectiveness is often measured differently by the patient (via symptom improvement) and by the healthcare provider (clinical lab tests). Outcome effectiveness for the same condition may be viewed differently by those performing the viewing. One healthcare provider may be happy with an A1C glucose level of 6.0 (American Diabetes Association Guidelines) while another is quite happy with 7.5 (because the level was previously over 12.0). The patient likely will not know *or care* whatsoever about the A1C glucose level. Both patient and healthcare provider are treating diabetes, yet each may have a different "effectiveness" threshold.

### ANTICIPATION

**Mammals love anticipation: Its emotional drives seem to be built, literally, into our DNA.** Anticipation requires a level of excitement and uneasiness about an action or path. The Gaming Industry is built on anticipation—the gambler pulling the lever of the slot machine, the spindles spinning round and round, excitement building, then the payday of the JackPot! More often than not, the repeat cycle with the next spin, is repeated over and over until success—or resignation. Win

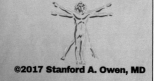

# ∼ CHAPTER 4: STRATEGY OVERVIEW ∽

or lose, either outcome has anticipation at its core. Gaming companies have mastered anticipation science.

All mammals, including human mammals, hate deprivation. We will go to great lengths to avoid or resolve deprivation. While some are more tolerant (Health Nuts) to deprivation, many (Food Rebels) are not. There must be an "end" in sight for any deprivation. The PrescriptFit Food Phases "prescribe" this deprivation as well as the relief. Moreover, patients chose their own level of deprivation and anticipation. While not a gamble, in the true sense of the word, PrescriptFit does satisfy gaming mantra—***our limits for deprivation are usually less than our limits of anticipation.*** In the PrescriptFit case, the JackPot is an improved symptom, a resolved disease, or pounds lost on the scale.

A patient may choose a 14-day plan for the quickest results and then find out their tolerance limit for each phase is 10 days, at which point they anticipate and "jump" to the next Phase. Unlike gambling, there is "no loser" with PrescriptFit. Symptoms and health measures improve, and you lose weight, albeit a little slower than expected, regardless of the degree of compliance.

## DISCOVERY

**We are a curious species—quite literally. We seem to always be looking for the next best thing.** PrescriptFit captures our curiosity by having patients "discover" how they feel (better symptoms), how they improve (lab tests), and how creative they can be with a food group (inventive). This combination makes PrescriptFit interesting. Being bored is not good for human success and productivity. PrescriptFit is not boring!

PRESCRIPTFIT®
MEDICAL NUTRITION THERAPY ▪ ▪ ▪ ▪ ▪ ▪ ▪

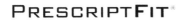

# SECTION B: DIVING IN...

*In Phase 8, you will add PrescriptFit® snacks, which will replace old, empty-calorie habits with nutritious snacks.*

## SURPRISE

**Engagement in activity is in direct proportion to the degree of surprise or joy we get from that activity.** Improvement of a miserable symptom, such as fatigue or heartburn, in three to five days is a joyful surprise. Watching your healthcare provider's face for a massively improved blood sugar measure is a joyful surprise (x 2: yours and your healthcare provider's). A sharply lower medication cost is a gleeful surprise, especially if the burden of multiple medications is keeping you strapped financially with little measurable benefit.

Even though I've been helping patients with nutrition therapy for over 30 years, I still get a great rush when my patient and I discover, with surprise, much improved life and hope for a healthy future that previously didn't exist!

## REINFORCEMENT

*It takes approximately three such successes and relapses for behavior to become ingrained enough to promote the healthier long-term diet strategy.*

**We all know about positive and negative reinforcement.** Both can steer behavior. PrescriptFit Food Phases are designed to amplify and focus behavior through measurable reinforcement. When a miserable symptom resolves without much deprivation and enjoyable taste, positive reinforcement occurs. The patient realizes, "I did this phase for X number of days and that misery, which was 10/10 a week ago, is now 3/10." When that same patient "Splurges" too often and for too prolonged a time frame, the symptoms return (often rapidly) to level 8/10. Then, the patient suffers a quite convincing negative reinforcement. Reinstituting the PrescriptFit strategy should immediately gain back improvement, giving yet more positive reinforcement and a strong lesson about cause and effect — the most powerful learning tool of all.

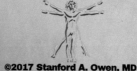

**PRESCRIPTFIT**®
MEDICAL NUTRITION THERAPY ▪ ▪ ▪ ▪ ▪ ▪ ▪

# CHAPTER 4: STRATEGY OVERVIEW

## EDUCATION

Our modern culture showers us with so many inexpensive food alternatives with fabulous taste presented in mixtures of nutrients and flavors, it is impossible to decipher if a particular product is causing harm. PrescriptFit Food Phase strategies help patients discover which food groups improve symptoms or provoke relapse. Using a perfect food (PrescriptFit products) to magnify improvement followed by simple, single food groups allows patients to self-discover how they feel and which measures improve. These are powerful educational experiences.

Most carbohydrates in our culture are mixed with fats or visa versa. Not until Dr. Atkins highlighted that fats, by themselves, are not as harmful as we believed, did anyone question the notion that food mixtures of fats and carbohydrates are different than either one eaten alone. Not until the science of cytokines exploded into mainstream medicine have we realized that Dr. Atkins' observations were not only correct, but the dieticians' probably were NOT!

## GROUP COHESION

**It is dangerous to not fit in! We are social animals and the "outsider" is a threat.** Anyone on a diet knows the feeling. PrescriptFit was designed to help everyone "fit in." Since no food groups are permanently excluded and all of the foods are accessible at any restaurant, PrescriptFit lets you easily dine out with family and friends. Only the first several Phases require eating differently than the norm.

Of those around you who may be hostile to changing your diet, family is likely the most hostile, followed by close friends then work colleagues.

*Each Phase includes tools and helpful hints for increasing your food options without compromising taste or your success:*

1. *The Grocery List — Find out what to buy for the companion recipes on www. drdiet.com as well as staples (such as seasonings) to help you create recipes that fit your and your family's needs. Grocery lists are included in Phases 1–8, when you are, perhaps, learning to experiment with new foods and recipes.*

2. *Taste tips — Brief notes on seasonings, spices, and how to use them to vary some of the basic recipes.*

3. *Sample recipes — Basic recipes for each phase can be found on www. drdiet.com.*

## PRESCRIPTFIT
MEDICAL NUTRITION THERAPY ▪ ▪ ▪ ▪ ▪ ▪ ▪

©2017 Stanford A. Owen, MD

# Section B: Diving In...

Those who ignore their immediate environment and social eating relationships struggle the greatest with long-term success. If one is a cocaine addict, it is not helpful to keep cocaine in the house! It is even more difficult if others in the house are also addicted. Cleaning up your food "environment" may be the most powerful approach to success.

## DISCIPLINE

**Knowledge combined with skill and then practiced over time = DISCIPLINE. Discipline is not a mental virtue but a system of operation.** Medicine is a discipline. Teaching is a discipline. Fire fighting is a discipline. All disciplines require a system of recording methods and outcomes.

PrescriptFit strategies make discipline very simple, literally 1—2—3. You only need to record what Food Phase you're using, how many minutes of exercise you performed, and if a "Splurge" occurred. It doesn't matter what was in your Splurge meal, ONLY that it is recorded with an asterix (*). Recording on paper, an APP, or some other device requires you to use your left, analytical brain. Analytical thinking is key to success. Hopeful thinking — the forte of your right brain — is emotional and incapable of solving problems. Interestingly, just the act of recording exercise, even if ZERO, is almost as powerful, predictably, as 30 minutes per day in achieving successful goals. This is because the ACT OF RECORDING is the discipline.

Medical Treatment

PrescriptFit®

Splurging

Healing & Education

PRESCRIPTFIT®
MEDICAL NUTRITION THERAPY ■ ■ ■ ■ ■ ■ ■

# ⇝ CHAPTER 4: STRATEGY OVERVIEW ⇝

## CHOICE/AUTONOMY

**Humans become violent without choice. We rebel. It is natural and normal.** Therefore, any diet that permanently restricts or removes a food item is doomed to incite rebellion and thus fail. PrescriptFit strategies allow you to Splurge twice a week (more or less) because that is what's necessary to avoid rebellion. The amount and type of food you splurge on are relatively unimportant. Our patients tell us that they need to be "socially acceptable" with Splurge foods twice per week.

Variety in food groups and methods of preparation will help you feel more satisfied and be more successful. For example, if you think grilled catfish can be the only item you would eat during Phase 2 (seafood), you're not realistically accounting for the variety that is surely part of your current life. Realistically, you will quickly tire of grilled catfish and will be tempted to find variety in something other than what is outlined in the Phase.

*We need to have fun occasionally. As the famous minstrel and songwriter Jimmy Buffett wrote of the occasional binge, "It cleans you out and then you can go on."*

## ARE YOU READY TO GET STARTED?

Now that you have some insight into the strategies behind this approach, let's take a tour of all 13 PrescriptFit Food Phases, starting with Food Phase 1 geared especially for medical treatment.

The "at-a-glance" diagram at right gives you an overview of how the food phases and how choice is built into the program.

| | Phase 1 | Amino Acids |
|---|---|---|
| **ALL YOU CAN EAT FROM EACH FOOD GROUP + 8 SERVINGS OF PRESCRIPTFIT AMINO ACIDS PER DAY** | Phase 2 | Seafood |
| | Phase 3 | Poultry |
| | Phase 4 | Vegetables |
| | Phase 5 | Eggs |
| | Phase 6 | Nuts |
| | Phase 7 | Fruit |
| | Phase 8 | PrescriptFit Snacks |
| **ALL YOU CAN EAT IN ONE "SPLURGE" MEAL - 8 ALLOWED PER MONTH** | Phase 9 | Pork |
| | Phase 10 | Beef |
| | Phase 11 | Caloric Beverages |
| | Phase 12 | Dairy |
| | Phase 13 | Starches |

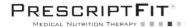

PRESCRIPTFIT
MEDICAL NUTRITION THERAPY ▪ ▪ ▪ ▪ ▪ ▪ ▪

# Section B: Diving In...

## Chapter 5: Medical Treatment with Amino Acids — Food Phase 1

No one likes to be told they're getting old or out of shape, but our metabolism will tell us the truth whether we like it or not! Obesity, age, and/or genetic predisposition often contribute to metabolic disorders. And many diseases related to diet have common genetic patterns. Recently, scientists have discovered new pieces of the metabolic puzzle related to fat cells, which:

> Produce abnormal proteins called cytokines that disturb metabolism

> Release cytokines into the bloodstream in response to the size and content of meals

> "Talk" constantly to the brain and other organs via the bloodstream and nerve fibers

The good news is that you can regulate the type of cytokine production by the amount of specific nutrition you feed your fat cells. That's exactly what Medical Nutrition Therapy (MNT) enables you to do. People who are sickest gain the most dramatic benefit. Even those expressing mild fatigue and "tiredness" are shocked at how much better they feel and how fast they improve.

## Why Your Old Diet Didn't Work for Long

Likely the way you have approached weight loss before has involved VLCD plans or approaches designed for quick weight loss. Long-term diet success can be safe and

Medical Treatment

PrescriptFit®

Splurging

Healing & Education

PRESCRIPTFIT®
MEDICAL NUTRITION THERAPY ▪ ▪ ▪ ▪ ▪ ▪ ▪

effective with VLCDs, but the changes you make in your eating habits need to be linked with feeling better and be sustainable for anyone in any family, work, and lifestyle situation. PrescriptFit focuses on getting well; weight loss is a bonus. The MNT Food Phase Strategy addresses the needs of reasonable people making reasonable progress towards being healthy and living longer.

*PrescriptFit is a food-based amino acid supplement that tastes great, is filling, and inexpensive — especially when compared to today's pharmaceutical and hospital costs.*

### PRESCRIPTFIT — VLCD AND BEYOND

PrescriptFit MNT starts with a VLCD strategy. A minimum of 800 calories (8 scoops) of PrescriptFit shakes, pudding, or soups meets minimum protein, carbohydrate, and calorie recommendations without medical supervision. Consuming only PrescriptFit products along with a complete multivitamin offers your body perfect nutrition — not just basic protein and carbohydrate, but a unique balance of micronized amino acids that optimize metabolism in the muscles, brain, and liver. The amino acid balance is especially helpful to cardiac muscle. Studies evaluating micronized amino acids in treatment of congestive heart failure in patients with diabetes reveal striking beneficial results.

A number of clinical benefits have been measured using PrescriptFit products in Phase 1 (VLCD) and are recorded in the PrescriptFit Calendar. Most patients record improvement in days measured on a 0–10 scale. Some of the key benefits recorded include:

> **Fatigue** — Patients experienced rapid improvement in fatigue symptoms (followed by breathlessness and heartburn).

> **Acid Heartburn** — 87 percent of PrescriptFit patients resolve acid heartburn without medication by week six.

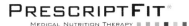

# SECTION B: DIVING IN...

> **Swelling (edema)** — This also responds very quickly, usually by day three and reaches peak fluid loss by week three.

> **Back and Joint Pain** — 63 percent of patients using pain medication for back and joint pain are able to discontinue medication by week 12.

> **Depression** — Symptoms of depression usually improve by week six.

> **Diabetes** — Virtually all program-compliant patients with diabetes improve blood glucose levels within days or weeks. Most require down-regulation of insulin and sulfonylurea (glyburide/glimepiride) medications; medical providers should remain vigilant with patients to decrease or discontinue such medicines. Those who have been on insulin for a decade or longer require longer periods of VLCD dieting to achieve remission without insulin.

These same symptoms and measures relapse with excessive Splurging. The difference from other diet plans is that, with the PrescriptFit Calendar score sheet, patients can easily correlate Splurging with misery, which motivates them to return quickly to the VLCD strategy again and again to relieve these symptoms. Instead of giving up, they realize that simply re-focusing on PrescriptFit strategies provides predictable, consistent relief.

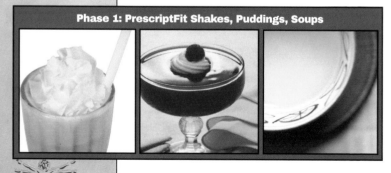

**Phase 1: PrescriptFit Shakes, Puddings, Soups**

**PRESCRIPTFIT**®
MEDICAL NUTRITION THERAPY ▪ ▪ ▪ ▪ ▪ ▪ ▪

# ⌐ CHAPTER 5: MEDICAL TREATMENT ⌐

## THE PRESCRIPTFIT ADVANTAGE

The PrescriptFit MNT Plan offers you multiple advantages over traditional diets:

> Amino acid supplements that regulate metabolism and banish cravings

> An easy-to-follow food plan that you can customize to your lifestyle

> Education and tools for long-term maintenance

> Measurable health improvements

You'll see results right from the start. Food Phase 1 of the PrescriptFit MNT Plan focuses on the amino acid supplements that provide complete nutrition as well as a satisfying taste and a feeling of fullness. Only the supplements are used for nutrition in Food Phase 1 (plus a daily multivitamin); no other food is allowed.

Depending on the rate at which you want to lose weight and/or improve symptoms, you can choose to stay on Food Phase 1 for three, seven, or 14 days. The longer you stay on this phase, the faster you may expect to see improvement.

If you are taking medications, you must ask your health care provider to monitor changes in your condition.

If you choose shorter Food Phase intervals (e.g., 3 days/Phase) yet do not achieve your weight or medical goals, simply repeat the 13 Food Phases at the same or longer intervals (e.g., 7 or 14 days/ Phase) until you achieve your goals.

PrescriptFit products are formulated using egg whites and nonfat milk solids and are fortified with additional branched-chain and **essential** amino acids: leucine, isoleucine, valine, lysine, histidine, and methionine in proprietary doses. Use of five or

*Every person can experience long-term diet success and good health, knowing that excessive Splurging (and fun) can be balanced immediately with PrescriptFit MNT products and strategies. This is a simple, logical, and nutritionally and socially acceptable method for any patient and every family.*

*"Essential" means the body cannot manufacture these amino acids from other dietary proteins.*

## PRESCRIPTFIT
MEDICAL NUTRITION THERAPY ▪ ▪ ▪ ▪ ▪ ▪

©2017 Stanford A. Owen, MD

# Section B: Diving In...

Be sure to take a daily multi-vitamin while using the PrescriptFit plan. If you were already taking vitamins or dietary supplements, you may continue to take them if your health practitioner agrees.

Make it easier to get started with PrescriptFit dosing by:

- Keeping your PrescriptFit product next to the blender at home or work.

- Taking one or several large thermos containers to work or in the car.

more doses guarantees a perfect balance of each amino acid per day. We recommend six doses as the minimum daily amount. Eight doses is optimal, but no overdose is possible. Twenty doses is the maximum recommended, even for those in strenuous exercise training programs. Do not take less than 6–8 doses per day during Food Phase 1 unless you are under a medical practitioner's care and supervision.

You'll find the exclusive use of PrescriptFit amino acid products in Food Phase 1 not only results in weight loss, symptom relief, and medical improvement, it also avoids confounding or confusing excuses for failure, such as Aunt Sue's pie or a bag of chips.

| PRESCRIPTFIT DAILY DOSING | |
| --- | --- |
| For Best Results | 6–8 doses (scoops) |
| To Maintain Your Success | 5+ doses (scoops) |
| Maximum Allowed (for strenuous exercise training programs) | 20 doses (scoops) |

Rather than sabotaging your success with extraneous foods, use Food Phase 1 to concentrate on how much and what medical measures (e.g., blood pressure, cholesterol, weight) and symptom measures (e.g., reduced pain, better sleep, more energy) begin to improve.

Some people ask, "What if I want to just stay with Phase 1 for an extended period of time?" If you have a more serious illness, you may continue use of amino acid supplements, without additional food, to normalize metabolic abnormalities as you adjust medication. Just be sure to continue to take a daily multivitamin and stay in close contact with your healthcare provider. If you use PrescriptFit products

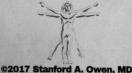

©2017 Stanford A. Owen, MD

# PRESCRIPTFIT
MEDICAL NUTRITION THERAPY ■ ■ ■ ■ ■ ■ ■

# CHAPTER 5: MEDICAL TREATMENT

exclusively for more than four weeks, please ask your healthcare provider to monitor your condition weekly.

PrescriptFit products come in a variety of flavors, all of which contain similar doses of branched-chain amino acids. You can alternate flavors through the day or week, or stick to one flavor, most commonly chocolate or vanilla, using different flavorings (listed on the next page) to provide variety during the week.

Supplement your PrescriptFit products with at least five, eight-ounce glasses of water or calorie-free beverages each day. You may even mix diet soft drinks with the PrescriptFit product (try Diet Coke or Diet Root Beer with the vanilla PrescriptFit to make a "float").

## AMINO ACIDS AS TREATMENT — MEASURING RESULTS

PrescriptFit products improve metabolism. You'll be able to measure results by symptom, physical, or laboratory improvement. As with any beneficial medication, PrescriptFit products can and should be used forever at five or more doses per day. If you discontinue the amino acids and resume the eating habits that originally caused the illness, symptoms will relapse.

If necessary, you can begin Food Phase 1 over again (and again, and again) if symptoms or diseases relapse and weight gain recurs. Relapse may occur with a particular food that you add during one of the Food Phases. Or, you may relapse months, even years later, if you revert to old eating habits. If this happens to you, simply go back to Food Phase 1 and start over, adding new Food Phases after control of your symptoms or conditions. If you responded the first time, you should respond again. With time and experience,

*PrescriptFit Flavors:*
- *Vanilla*
- *Chocolate*
- *Chicken and Beef Soups*
- *Lactose-Free Vanilla or Chocolate (for making puddings and for those susceptible to gas and diarrhea from ingestion of milk (lactose).*

*Patients with Irritable Bowel Syndrome (IBS) improve markedly using the Lactose-Free products (for more information on IBS, see pages 167–169).*

*Optimal results occur when PrescriptFit shakes or soups are used prior to or with a meal in future Food Phases.*

PRESCRIPTFIT
MEDICAL NUTRITION THERAPY

©2017 Stanford A. Owen, MD

# SECTION B: DIVING IN...

## THE GROCERY LIST

This "Grocery List" offers possible products you can add to PrescriptFit products. After Phase 1, you can use your imagination – if it doesn't contain fat or sugar, you can add it!

### ADDITIVES FLAVORINGS PUDDING MIXES

- Jell-O™-Brands (Sugar-free only)

- Watkins™ specialty flavorings and herbs

- Spices (cinnamon, pumpkin pie, nutmeg)

- McCormick™ flavorings

- Crystal Light® soft drinks

- Tea or coffee — Mix sugar substitute, PrescriptFit vanilla flavor, and a bit of water for coffee creamer

you'll recognize the food category culprit(s) contributing to relapse, and you'll learn to avoid them.

### TASTE TIPS: ADDING FLAVOR, VARIETY, COLOR, AND TEXTURE TO PRESCRIPTFIT PRODUCTS

You'll want to experiment with adding a variety of sugar-free flavorings to your PrescriptFit products. Remember, variety will prevent boredom and encourage your continued success with the Food Phase plan. If you experience demonstrable health improvements using PrescriptFit products, you'll want to continue them forever, but not if you're bored. Your "Grocery List" (at left) lists possible additives. In Food Phase 7, add fresh, canned, or frozen fruit to your shakes for a real treat. Avoid canned or frozen fruit preserved with sugar.

### To obtain optimal flavor:

> Fill the glass or cup with ice and/or water first. Add 1–3 scoops of PrescriptFit (1 for a small cup, 3 for a large glass). Blend for 2 minutes for a creamy shake, 1 minute for an icy shake.

> PrescriptFit shakes will stay blended (hot or cold) in a thermos.

> PrescriptFit amino acids are stable when frozen or heated. For great treats and desserts (especially for kids, teens) use wooden sticks and plastic popsicle molds for frozen treats. Try chocolate and Crystal Light flavorings.

> For a thicker shake, add additional powder, more ice, and blend for a longer time so that the egg whites will cause the product to "soufflé" into a creamy delight.

> Hot drinks (hot chocolate and soups) are best blended first in hot water. Prolonged microwave heating may result in coagulation of the egg whites. Experiment with timing.

PRESCRIPTFIT®
MEDICAL NUTRITION THERAPY ▪ ▪ ▪ ▪ ▪ ▪ ▪

# ⚬ CHAPTER 5: MEDICAL TREATMENT ⚬

## LORETTA — A FAMILY SUCCESS STORY

When Loretta came to the clinic, she was a 40-year-old mother of three teenage boys and had gained 35 pounds with each pregnancy and an additional 20 pounds since the youngest was born 13 years ago. At 280 pounds, she now suffered from diabetes, hypertension, severe back and knee pain, and was constantly exhausted due to sleep apnea. Out of "love" for her children, Loretta has denied no foods or snacks to the entire family. Consequently, all but one child (and her husband) are substantially overweight.

Loretta was referred by her healthcare provider, who gave her less than five years to live if she didn't get her health and diet under control. After a lengthy discussion about the difficulty and commitment necessary to lose 130 pounds and some problem solving with the dietician, it was decided she would prepare meals from Phase 1–8 for her children while using the 14-day per Phase plan (a total of 26 weeks to complete all 13 Phases). Her boys could use shakes and snacks as desired. The family reluctantly agreed to remove all snacks and calorie-laden drinks from the house, including milk and juice (two "sleeper" obesity-causing beverages). The PrescriptFit shakes have ample calcium, even for growing boys. She bought an ample supply of snack bars and shakes to prevent anyone in the family from feeling deprived.

Loretta practiced recipes from each of the first eight Phases for most meals and prepared two "splurge" meals per week for the entire family, usually mid-week and on Sunday. This prepared Loretta conceptually and practically for each Phase. On Saturday, her kids went out with friends for pizza or burgers.

Her husband bought her a stationary bicycle with arm attachments, a used treadmill, and exercise ball for less than $500, which she used every morning. He agreed to walk with her every afternoon for 15 minutes or longer. She rarely recorded less than 30 minutes of exercise per day on her PrescriptFit Calendar.

Loretta achieved complete remission of her diabetes within two weeks (never to return), discontinued blood pressure medication by four weeks, resolved her back and knee pain by 12 weeks, and lost a total of 140 pounds. Her family collectively lost 70 pounds (husband lost 40 and the kids lost about 10 pounds each).

The total cost of the weight loss Phases was less than the medication cost and medical visits of only the prior six months (just her insurance deductible, not the actual cost). With good planning, open communication, and love, Loretta and her family were successful.

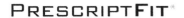

# PRESCRIPTFIT
MEDICAL NUTRITION THERAPY ■ ■ ■ ■ ■ ■ ■

# SECTION B: DIVING IN...

## PHASE 1 RECIPES — DOSING AND MIXING

### SHAKES: Vanilla or Chocolate (regular or lactose-free)

1. Add 1–4 scoops of PrescriptFit amino acid powder to 4–5 ounces of water in a blender.

2. Add several cubes of ice (and/or water) and blend. Continue to add powder and/or ice to reach desirable thickness, taste, and texture. Some like crunchy ice shakes; others prefer smooth and thick shakes like those from fast-food restaurants. The most important point is to experiment with how you like your product to taste. There is no limit or quantity of PrescriptFit powder to each shake. Remember to use 6–8 doses (scoops) per day in Food Phases 1–13.

3. To boost flavor, simple add your favorite spice or flavoring toward the end of blending.

**PUDDINGS** — Lactose-free Chocolate and Vanilla make perfect puddings in 30 seconds! Plus, these quick clean-up treats are great for those on the go.

1. Place 1–3 doses (scoops) in a cup or bowl.

2. Drizzle in water while stirring until the desired texture of pudding is reached.

3. For variety, add spices, nuts (Phase 5), or nonfat whipped cream (Phase 12).

**SOUPS** — The chicken and beef soups are spicy, but you can mix them to suit your taste.

1. Start with 1 cup of hot water and mix (with a whisk) or blend.

2. Add ½ scoop when first mixing and another ½ scoop until you like the taste. Mixing one scoop of Beef Soup with one scoop of Chicken Soup produces a delightful blend.

**Now you're ready for the Education and Healing Phases of PrescriptFit MNT.**

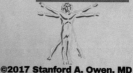

**PRESCRIPTFIT**®
MEDICAL NUTRITION THERAPY ▪ ▪ ▪ ▪ ▪ ▪ ▪

# CHAPTER 6: HEALING & EDUCATION — PHASES 2–8

## PHASE 2 SEAFOOD

Seafood is one of nature's most perfect foods, especially for those with chronic medical conditions related to diet. Seafood is virtually 100 percent protein and contains minimal fat, with the exception of certain fish (tuna, salmon, sardines, mullet, mackerel) that contain Omega 3 fatty acids, which are beneficial to the cardiovascular system and brain. Due to the low-calorie content of seafood, it is virtually impossible to "overdose" on seafood and gain weight unless large amounts of butter or oil are mixed with the fish.

Seafood is satiating because protein does not stimulate hunger-causing insulin, takes longer to digest, and tastes great. Seafood does not stimulate toxic cytokines.

However, seafood does not contain essential vitamins found in vegetables or fruit; therefore, vitamin supplementation is essential if a "seafood only" diet is utilized with PrescriptFit amino acids.

## SEAFOOD MYTHS

**Cholesterol** — Shellfish contain cholesterol-like molecules (sterols). For years, scientists thought that seafood elevated cholesterol levels or would be harmful to those with cholesterol blockage that cause heart attack or stroke. Seafood-only diets can lower cholesterol in most patients, often dramatically. You and your healthcare provider can test this by measuring cholesterol levels at the end of Food Phase 1 and again at the end of Food Phase 2.

*Seafood Choices: Fish (fresh or saltwater), Shrimp, Crab, Lobster, Crawfish, Oysters, Mussels, Clams*

**PRESCRIPTFIT**
MEDICAL NUTRITION THERAPY ▪ ▪ ▪ ▪ ▪ ▪ ▪

©2017 Stanford A. Owen, MD

# SECTION B: DIVING IN...

*Check with your local Fish and Wildlife Department regarding fish caught in local streams. Most states check toxin levels in local seafood.*

**Toxins** — But what about the mercury and other toxins reportedly found in seafood? Magazine articles have noted mercury, cadmium, and dioxin (PCBs) found in different fish populations. However, levels are usually present at concentrations that are medically insignificant. Only farm-raised salmon from Europe have been found with PCB levels that could be a risk if you ate it daily for years or decades. European fish are raised with bait fish caught in more polluted waters of the North and Baltic Seas. Toxin levels are not significant for North or South American farm-raised salmon.

*Avoid eating raw seafood if you have liver or immune disease, you are being treated with chemotherapy, or if you take antacid medication.*

Bacteria are present in some shellfish, especially oysters and clams. Vibrio species of bacteria are common in salt marshes and are not contaminants, but rather, normal marsh inhabitants. Raw shellfish might contain sufficient numbers of bacteria to cause symptoms (diarrhea). Individuals with liver or immune disease (on chemotherapy) should not eat raw seafood. Those taking antacid medication should also avoid raw shellfish, as stomach acid kills most bacteria inhabiting shellfish. Except for steaming, all other forms of cooking destroy the bacteria. A few cases of bacterial dysentery have been reported in steamed lobsters. Horseradish used to dip raw oysters has been shown to kill shellfish bacteria. Shellfish-related diarrhea is rare.

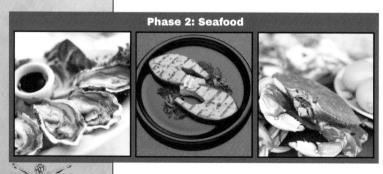

**Phase 2: Seafood**

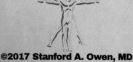

**PRESCRIPTFIT**®
MEDICAL NUTRITION THERAPY ▪ ▪ ▪ ▪ ▪ ▪ ▪

# CHAPTER 6: HEALING & EDUCATION

## SEAFOOD AND CALORIES

Seafood is the best calorie "bang for your buck" at 25 calories per ounce (35 per ounce for fatty fishes). This means that one pound (16 ounces) of seafood is only 400 calories if cooked without fat or oil. Since you would have to eat more calories than you burn to gain weight, it is virtually impossible to gain weight on non-fried or non-sautéed seafood.

## CATEGORIES OF SEAFOOD — ARE THERE DIFFERENCES?

Are there nutritional and caloric differences between types of seafood? What about shellfish vs. fish? Yes there are differences, but practically speaking, the differences are not significant enough to cause concern. Fatty fish are higher in Omega 3 fats and have slightly more calories. These few extra calories are insignificant to weight gain and may be offset by health benefits. We recommend using seafood in Food Phase 2 because seafood tastes great, is filling, has few calories per serving, and contains no nutrients that induce abnormal chemistry.

Variety is important to keep interest, prevent boredom, or cause aversion. Using different types of seafood in Food Phase 2 will likely make seafood more desirable. Experiment!

## WHAT IF I CAN'T OR WON'T EAT SEAFOOD?

If you are allergic to seafood, you may use poultry or vegetables in Phase 2. Or, you can substitute nonfat cottage cheese. Be sure to read the directions for Food Phase 3 (Poultry) or Food Phase 4 (Vegetables) or Food Phase 12 (Dairy) before you begin. Vegetarian? No problem. Simply skip the seafood, poultry, beef, and pork Phases. Remember, the PrescriptFit product, with a multivitamin is PERFECT food. Everything else is entertainment.

### IMPOSSIBLE TO GAIN ON SEAFOOD

It takes 11 calories/pound/day for the average woman (12 for a man) to maintain weight. Those numbers represent your Basal Metabolic Rate (BMR).

Subtract one calorie/pound/day from your total metabolism at age 40 and again at age 65 since metabolism naturally slows with age. Using these calculations, consider the following example:

To gain 1 pound of fat, a 160-pound, 40 year-old woman would need to consume 5,100 calories, of which 1,600 could be for maintenance (10 calories/day X 160 pounds = BMR) and 3,500 would represent the energy needed for one pound of fat.

Thus, she would need to eat 13 pounds of seafood (5,100 calories divided by 400 calories/pound) to gain 1 pound in a given day! She would need to eat 5 pounds per day to gain one pound in a week.

Not likely!

PRESCRIPTFIT
MEDICAL NUTRITION THERAPY ▪ ▪ ▪ ▪ ▪ ▪ ▪

©2017 Stanford A. Owen, MD

# Section B: Diving In...

Fried or sautéed seafood contains 125 calories/ounce compared to 25 calories/ounce for seafood prepared without oil. Oil contains 125 calories/ level tablespoon. Remember that 1 mile of walking burns 100 calories. Thus, frying and sautéing seafood requires 1 mile of walking to pay for the calories in only 1 ounce of fried seafood.

For mouth-watering seafood recipes, view the Recipe section at www.drdiet.com.

## Methods of Cooking Seafood

Seafood meat is flaky and porous compared to a steak. You can break off little pieces of cooked fish with a fork, which you could not do with a piece of steak. This means that the meat fibers of fish are able to soak up oil. In fact, fish cooked in oil or butter will soak up enough oil to equal the same caloric value of fatty red meat. Red meat on the other hand is already saturated with fat and therefore cannot soak up additional oil.

With these facts in mind, you'll want to avoid fried or sautéed fish (unless used as a "splurge" meal). Instead, boil, poach, broil, steam, bake, or grill your seafood. The PrescriptFit recipes will help you use stocks and flavorings to achieve better flavor from sautéed fish.

The most common "mistake" when preparing flavorful seafood is over cooking. You needn't worry about cooking fish to a "safe" temperature since raw fish is safe to eat (if fresh). Fatty fish is especially vulnerable to over cooking. The oil in the fish changes flavor when it is heated. Therefore, cooked tuna or salmon tastes radically different than slightly browned fish with a pink center.

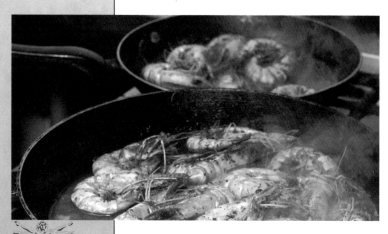

**PRESCRIPTFIT**®
MEDICAL NUTRITION THERAPY ■ ■ ■ ■ ■ ■ ■

# CHAPTER 6: HEALING & EDUCATION

## SHOPPING FOR SEAFOOD

Often, people are wary of buying seafood simply because they don't know what to buy or what to look for. Here are some simple tips:

1. Buy fresh from a fish market if possible.
2. If you buy from a supermarket, buy frozen fish. Do not buy the fish from a display case. The seafood is almost always previously frozen and thawed in the store unless it is specifically marked "fresh caught."
3. When buying frozen seafood, buy sealed bags. Look for bags with little or no ice crystals in the bag.
4. Thaw the fish, in its bag, in a bowl of room temperature water. Rinse the fish once thawed. It is then ready to cook.

Use shopping to reinforce your Food Phase strategies. If you buy seafood from the supermarket, go directly to the seafood section when beginning your shopping, since seafood is the first "food" Phase of the PrescriptFit Plan. From the seafood section, go directly to poultry (Food Phase 3), then vegetables (Food Phase 4). Strategic shopping will reinforce strategic diet planning.

### Dosing

*There is no health or weight-gain restriction on the amount or type of seafood allowable per day on the PrescriptFit MNT plan. All you can eat!*

---

## DEVON — NEW WAYS TO ENJOY SEAFOOD

Devon grew up in the Mississippi Delta. She never ate seafood that was not fried. The thought of baked fish made her nauseated. Her usual experience with poultry was either fried by her grandmother, or usually, from a fast food establishment. Even the Thanksgiving turkey is fried and injected with butter.

Willing to keep an open mind, Devon's husband started preparing seafood on the barbecue pit. They then experimented with PrescriptFit recipes (some of which have been used in a national television cooking program). Over a period of several years, both Devon and her husband became fans of PrescriptFit food preparation. They still eat fried foods but on "splurge" meals twice a week or less.

**CASE STUDY**

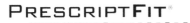

# PRESCRIPTFIT
MEDICAL NUTRITION THERAPY ▪ ▪ ▪ ▪ ▪ ▪ ▪

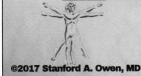

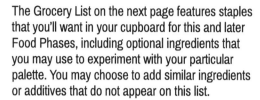

# SECTION B: DIVING IN...

The Grocery List on the next page features staples that you'll want in your cupboard for this and later Food Phases, including optional ingredients that you may use to experiment with your particular palette. You may choose to add similar ingredients or additives that do not appear on this list.

You will notice that several herbs and fresh garlic are used to season the dishes we feature at www.drdiet.com. These ingredients are approved for this phase as a seasoning. Feel free to experiment; just remember that all flavor additives must meet the requirement of being sugar-free and fat-free.

Discover numerous simple and delicious methods for preparing seafood that allow you to enjoy what you are eating without foregoing taste.

## BOB OWEN'S SEAFOOD RECIPES

Bob Owen has earned legendary status among friends and family for his uncanny sense of balance when merging tastes through herbs, cooking technique, and food combinations.

He had two recipes "retired" into the legendary category in famous chef Bobby Flay's library after a single appearance on Flay's television show. Both recipes he invented for the show and had never been prepared previously. Genius is born, not made.

Enjoy a small sampling of Bob's abilities by visiting the Recipe section at www.drdiet.com

- Skillet Lemon Fish
- Lemon Garlic Shrimp
- Seared White Fish
- Baked Black Pepper Fish or Shrimp
- Dill, Rosemary & Sage Salmon
- Cracked Black Pepper Seared Tuna Steak

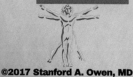

**PRESCRIPTFIT**®
MEDICAL NUTRITION THERAPY ▪ ▪ ▪ ▪ ▪ ▪ ▪

# ∽ CHAPTER 6: HEALING & EDUCATION ∽

## THE GROCERY LIST

*Stock your pantry with the ingredients below for creating tasty seafood (Phase 2) and poultry (Phase 3) recipes:*

- Chicken broth or chicken bouillon cubes (soft variety preferred)
- Beef broth
- Fat-free butter spray or Benecol® butter
- Butter powder (Butter Buds® or Molly McButter® powder found in the seasoning aisle)
- Black pepper, white pepper, Crushed red peppers
- Salt, sea salt, kosher salt
- Cajun/Creole seasoning mix or red pepper seasoning mix
- Blackening seasoning (If available)
- Non-stick cooking spray
- Garlic powder, chili powder
- Balsamic Vinegar
- Worcestershire sauce
- Tony Chachere's™ seasoning mix
- Lemons or lemon juice (fresh lemon juice highly suggested)
- Chopped or minced garlic
- Chives and onions
- Fresh or dried herbs, such as Dill, Parsley, Sage, Thyme, Oregano, Cilantro, Bay leaves and Basil
- Jalapeño peppers
- Capers
- Leeks
- Optional: PrescriptFit Chicken Soup for gravy

*If you like butter flavor, use Benecol™ or Smart Balance™ artificial butter made from plant stanols. These products lower cholesterol and triglycerides almost as much as cholesterol medication and improve artery function. They also taste great.*

*PrescriptFit Chicken and Beef Soup supplements provide excellent taste to enhance flavor as well as daily protein requirements and branched-chain amino acids.*

*Although there are no restrictions on the amount of seafood you eat, several ingredients commonly used when preparing seafood are excluded from Phase 2, including flour, cornmeal, bread crumbs, and most store-bought batter.*

## PRESCRIPTFIT®
MEDICAL NUTRITION THERAPY ▪ ▪ ▪ ▪ ▪ ▪ ▪

# SECTION B: DIVING IN...

## PHASE 3 POULTRY

Poultry is your next logical addition to the PrescriptFit MNT Plan because, like seafood, poultry is inexpensive, filling, low in calories, versatile, tastes great, and does not provoke cytokine production. Though you may choose to substitute poultry for seafood, poultry typically follows seafood since the fat content is higher and, therefore, the calorie content is higher.

Like seafood, there are no restrictions on the amount of poultry you eat; however, the same ingredients commonly used when preparing poultry are excluded from Phase 3 (e.g., flour, cornmeal, bread crumbs).

## POULTRY AS NUTRITION

Poultry contains no carbohydrate. Poultry muscle is quite lean, containing minimal amounts of fat. Most of the fat content of poultry, which is saturated, harmful fat, is contained in the skin on the surface of the muscle. Both the skin and surface fat should be removed before cooking.

Poultry contains about 50 calories/ounce (seafood is 25 calories/ounce) due to the increased fat content. Leaving the skin on brings the calorie/ounce to about 75–100, depending on how much drainage is allowed during cooking. An

**Phase 3: Poultry**

## PRESCRIPTFIT®
MEDICAL NUTRITION THERAPY ▪ ▪ ▪ ▪ ▪ ▪ ▪

average breast weighs about 4 ounces, or 200 calories without the skin. Leaving the skin on not only raises the calorie count to around 300–400 calories, it also adds saturated fat, which provokes cytokines along with adverse effects on insulin, cortisone, and lipid (cholesterol) metabolism.

Poultry protein is high in the amino acid tryptophan. Tryptophan can cause sedation and may be responsible for the "coma" or excessive tired feeling that follows a typical Thanksgiving meal of turkey. However, by Food Phase 3 most people are feeling so much more energized that any sedating effect from poultry is minimal. Do be on the lookout for sedating effects that become uncomfortable. If excessive sedation is a problem, use poultry sparingly.

As with any meat, poultry is filling and satiating. The protein takes longer to digest and does not vigorously stimulate insulin unless a large amount of chicken fat is consumed. Like seafood, poultry is deficient in certain vitamins. Continuation of a multivitamin is mandatory.

## POULTRY TOXIN MYTHS

The U.S. Food and Drug Administration has scrutinized poultry producers for the commercial use of artificial hormones and phosphates to enhance growth. No definite link to human disease has been documented. Most modern poultry farms do not add toxic products to the feed, and many progressive growing houses are using natural feed devoid of hormones or growth-producing nutrients.

"Free Range" chicken is very lean and tastes different from commercially raised chicken. Range-fed chickens can quit feeding when they are not hungry or when the work of finding food is more uncomfortable than the hunger. Range chicken is preferable if available and affordable.

> You must remove the skin and visible fat before cooking your poultry. You'll find many appealing ways to prepare poultry without adding a lot of calories and fat!

> REMEMBER SATURATED FAT PROVOKES CYTOKINES!

> "Free Range" chicken is a term used to described chicken raised "the old fashioned way" in the barnyard or fields, either pecking a meal from grass seeds or being fed grain by the local farmer.

PRESCRIPTFIT
MEDICAL NUTRITION THERAPY ▪ ▪ ▪ ▪ ▪ ▪ ▪

©2017 Stanford A. Owen, MD

# SECTION B: DIVING IN...

## CATEGORIES OF POULTRY — CHICKEN, TURKEY, DUCK, QUAIL, PHEASANT, OTHER BIRDS

There are differences between different birds and differences among same bird species depending on how the birds are raised and fed (keep in mind human analogies). All birds fed "naturally" are leaner and contain less fat. "Naturally" means as they would feed and exercise in nature: searching for food; finding only lean food; resting when full; running from enemies; chasing mates; and defending territory from intruders. Imagine how much easier it would be to keep your weight under control if you live "naturally!" Chickens confined to a small space in a chicken factory cannot move (exercise), are bored (no "playground" interaction), and are constantly exposed to high-fat feed. No wonder they are fatter than range chickens! Sound familiar to human obesity?

Duck is most capable of accumulating fat when fed excessively. Therefore, domestic duck is quite high in calories (100 calories/ounce unless stripped completely of fat). If you ever roast duck, you will notice a large puddle of grease in the pot after cooking. Wild duck is nonfat, even with the skin, and tastes nothing like domestic duck. Wild duck requires prolonged cooking with many herbs (see recipes) for palatability.

Chicken is next most fat. Turkey is quite lean. Since turkeys are difficult to keep penned in confined space like chickens, they get some exercise.

Pheasant and quail are quite lean, especially if wild. Ostrich and emus are large birds that are raised commercially but have not caught on as inexpensive food sources. These two birds are quite lean for the same reasons as turkey—they are too large to confine and must be "range" fed.

©2017 Stanford A. Owen, MD

# PRESCRIPTFIT®
MEDICAL NUTRITION THERAPY ▪ ▪ ▪ ▪ ▪ ▪ ▪

# CHAPTER 6: HEALING & EDUCATION

## SAFELY STORING POULTRY

As you may know, poultry is easily contaminated with bacteria. As with humans, animals kept in a confined space with common handlers spread germs by proximity. At slaughter, these bacteria are transmitted through fecal material. Salmonella, the most common organism found contaminating poultry, causes intestinal disease with diarrhea. Careless handling of intestine in the butchering process can spread the disease. Some studies found 40 percent of chicken meat tested positive for salmonella. While community rates of diarrhea are lower than 40 percent, play it safe and assume your meat is contaminated. Poison-producing E. coli bacteria also has been found in chicken. Here are some tips for safely handling poultry:

> Always store poultry in the refrigerator until ready to cook.

> Thaw frozen poultry in the refrigerator or in the microwave just before cooking.

### Dosing

*No portion or dose restrictions are used for poultry. All you can eat. Enjoy!*

### SAM — FINDING A WORKING BALANCE

Sam had been diagnosed with sleep apnea, severe fatigue, and high blood pressure when he began the PrescriptFit MNT Plan. He became symptom-free (no fatigue), abolished snoring, and normalized blood pressure without medication after completing Food Phase 2 (seafood + amino acids) of the Plan (4 weeks). Within one week of adding Food Phase 3 (poultry), his wife noticed increased snoring, and Sam reported fatigue to a level one-half his initial experience.

He admitted using large amounts of poultry and minimal seafood the first week into Food Phase 3. I had him return to Food Phase 2 for one week, then resume Food Phase 3 with limited amounts (one meal/day) of poultry. His snoring and fatigue completely resolved when he resumed Food Phase 2 and did not return with the limited poultry when re-starting Food Phase 3.

Sam had no further problems with Food Phase 4 (vegetables) or beyond.

CASE STUDY

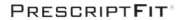

PRESCRIPTFIT
MEDICAL NUTRITION THERAPY ▪ ▪ ▪ ▪ ▪ ▪ ▪

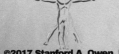

©2017 Stanford A. Owen, MD

# SECTION B: DIVING IN...

*As a rule, poultry is much more tender if cooked in a broth, gravy, or stew than if cooked on a grill or dry in an oven. Nevertheless, low heat, slow cooking, or slow smoking is a fantastic means of retaining the tenderness of the poultry while adding flavor. Just be sure to monitor for tenderness while cooking.*

> Don't eat undercooked poultry! Use a meat thermometer, and make sure it registers 180 degrees (170 degrees for breast meat) before you stop cooking it.

Feel free to experiment; just remember that all flavor additives must be sugar-free and fat-free additions. My best advice for your poultry experiments: Don't limit your options. Yet, until you become familiar with new seasonings, you'd be wise to add small amounts of seasoning at a time. This is especially true of the more pungent herbs, such as cilantro, anise or fennel seed, or spices like red or white pepper.

If you're dreaming of crispy, greasy, fried chicken, wake up! No fried foods are allowed, except for "splurge" meals, during the PrescriptFit MNT Plan.

## CHARLEY & HIS WIFE — THEIR PRESCRIPTFIT SOLUTION

Charley is a meat eater. He could eat meat or follow the Atkins diet forever. His wife, on the other hand, hates meat. She is borderline vegetarian and loves pasta. Charley blames his wife's pasta and bread on his beer-belly physique. The two compromised: Charley would use the barbecue grill as often as possible to prepare seafood, poultry, and meat dishes while grilling vegetables. He was responsible for being creative with the veggies. Much to his surprise (and his wife's), Charley became enthralled with vegetable and meat dishes.

It soon became apparent that, indeed, his wife's addiction to carbs was an issue. Since they agreed to "splurging" two meals per week, she was forced to consider other carb-like foods.

She focused on dessert dishes made with PrescriptFit products and snack bars to make up the sweet/carb cravings. He remained a meat-a-holic with a vegetarian flare. While their basic food instincts were not changed (they rarely do), their style developed individual characteristics. Most marriage weight gain is similar to Charley and his wife: trying to "eat together" with different preferences and styles—a sure path to weight gain.

**CASE STUDY**

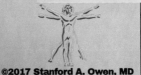

**PRESCRIPTFIT**®
MEDICAL NUTRITION THERAPY ▪ ▪ ▪ ▪ ▪ ▪

# ⌁ CHAPTER 6: HEALING & EDUCATION ⌁

Like fish, poultry meat is more porous and "stringy" than beef and can accumulate oil when frying or basting in its own grease. Like fish, poultry will accumulate enough oil when fried to equal caloric content of beef at 125 calories/ounce, over twice the calories as non-fried poultry prepared without the skin (grilled, baked, broiled, boiled, or stewed in broth). If you're craving fried chicken, save it for one of your eight "splurge" meals per month allowed in Food Phase 9 and beyond.

You'll discover delicious, new ways to prepare poultry. Poultry makes excellent soups with relative ease by combining chicken broth and chicken bouillon cubes, which taste similar to a homemade stock. You can also make gravy by combining broth, bouillon and PrescriptFit Chicken Soup. Finally, anyone can make a low-fat, low-calorie butter flavor sauce by combining chicken broth, bouillon and butter flavored powder, such as Butter Buds® or Molly McButter®.

Because poultry is a popular source of protein throughout the world, there are many styles of cooking poultry. You may want to experiment with regional flavor combinations to develop a distinctive dish. For example, if you want to make Italian style chicken, use typical Italian ingredients such as basil, oregano, thyme, sage, and garlic. Or, if you want to cook a Cajun style dish, use red and black pepper, garlic, onion powder, celery salt, etc. All seasonings are acceptable as long as they do not add sugar or fat to the recipe.

Remember: The most important aspect of the PrescriptFit MNT program is the amino acid supplement. Make sure that you are consuming the correct amount of doses for your plan.

---

### BOB OWEN'S POULTRY RECIPES

- Chicken Soup
- Baked Chicken (Pieces and Whole)
- Blackened Chicken
- Braised Garlic and Green Onion Chicken

*To access these and other great recipes, visit the recipe section at www.drdiet.com*

*Get started preparing tasty poultry dishes.*

---

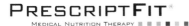

PRESCRIPT FIT®
MEDICAL NUTRITION THERAPY ▪ ▪ ▪ ▪ ▪ ▪ ▪

©2017 Stanford A. Owen, MD

# Section B: Diving In...

## Phase 4 Vegetables

Vegetables are added to the early phases of the PrescriptFit MNT Plan because they are low in calories and simple sugar, high in filling fiber, and loaded with vitamins, minerals, antioxidants, and phytonutrients.

### Vegetables as Nutrition

Vegetables enhance blood vessel function, fight cancer, and balance intestinal bacteria colonies. Vegetables can be used to enhance the flavor of the amino acid supplements as well as the seafood and chicken recipes from Food Phases 2–3. Vegetables provide an endless variety of color, texture, smell, taste, and nutrition. Vegetables are filling.

Unlimited amounts of vegetables on the Phase 4 list are allowed in Food Phase 4 of the PrescriptFit MNT Plan. However, starchy vegetables (corn, potatoes, peas, dried beans, winter squash) are reserved for Food Phase 13. The larger carbohydrate load added by starchy vegetables could induce insulin resistance, cause a relapse of symptoms, and promote weight gain. If you crave starchy vegetables, you'll be better off saving them for a splurge meal after you've achieved significant improvement and weight loss.

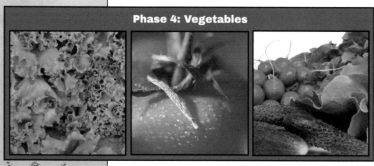

Phase 4: Vegetables

PRESCRIPTFIT®
MEDICAL NUTRITION THERAPY ■ ■ ■ ■ ■ ■ ■

# CHAPTER 6: HEALING & EDUCATION

Food Phase 4 of the PrescriptFit MNT plan recommends five or more servings of vegetables per day, along with 6–8 doses of amino acids, and as much seafood or poultry as desired. At the very least, include a vegetable serving at breakfast, lunch, and supper. If you combine two servings at lunch and dinner with one serving for breakfast, you'll meet your five-a-day requirement.

## VEGETABLE MYTHS

Many people are convinced that consumption of vegetable extracts, squeezed vegetable juices, and huge doses of vitamins will bring health or prevent disease. The public buys and consumes these products every day at staggering costs, never suspecting there is a better, safer, less-expensive way to enjoy the benefits of vegetables.

Most of the benefits of herbal products were extrapolated from the evidence that people consuming diets very high in vegetable content were spared many chronic illnesses associated with obesity. Whole vegetables (and fruit) behave much differently in the human intestine than juiced, dried, or concentrated portions of those vegetables. Bacteria in the intestine grow on vegetable fiber, vegetable nutrients, and vegetable sugars. The bacteria produce chemicals that increase anticancer immune function. By using purified products, the benefits of whole vegetables might well be missed.

Eating five servings or more of diverse vegetables per day assures vitamin, mineral, and intestinal bacterial balance. An ideal strategy is to consume five different colors of vegetables daily: green, yellow, purple, red, or orange. Each color:

> Represents different phytonutrients, vitamins, minerals, and plant sugars.

> Adds different flavor and variety

**Dosing**

*There is no portion or dose restriction with non-starchy vegetables. Eat as much as you desire — the more the better.*

*Remember — variety prevents boredom. You've read this over and over in this book; it should be your mantra by now!*

PRESCRIPTFIT
MEDICAL NUTRITION THERAPY ■ ■ ■ ■ ■ ■ ■

©2017 Stanford A. Owen, MD

# SECTION B: DIVING IN...

## ORGANIC VEGETABLES

Debate has raged for years over the health implications of organically grown vegetables versus traditional commercial farming methods. "Organic" vegetables are grown without pesticide, without artificial growth-enhancing chemicals or fertilizers, and are not shipped with preservative chemicals. Proponents claim organic vegetables contain more minerals, vitamins, and nutrients.

Buy organic produce if you prefer. But, keep in mind that your food choices should be realistic and truly pertinent to your health; avoiding vegetables because organic options are either not available or are more expensive probably isn't a healthy choice.

## CALORIES & VEGETABLE CATEGORIES

Vegetables, including starchy ones (corn, dried beans, potatoes), are the lowest calorie food per unit of any food group. Vegetables are even lower in calories, by weight, than seafood because vegetables are high in non-digestible fiber and low in sugar. Vegetables are bulky and filling.

We measure vegetables by the cup. To visualize one cup, try this experiment: chop any type of vegetable, place into a measuring cup, then pour the contents onto a dinner plate. Note the large volume on the dinner plate. Make a mental note how few calories per cup fill up that plate.

Vegetables differ in calorie content by the amount of carbohydrate, fat, and fiber they contain. Most vegetables have relatively small amounts of fat or protein. Green, leafy vegetables are very low in calories, while starchy vegetables have the highest caloric content – 200 calories per cup. One cup of beans will almost cover a dinner plate; yet it contains less calories than two bites of a fatty steak.

The table on the next page features the main vegetable categories by calorie. Remember, for any food, you must walk one mile at 100 calories per mile to "pay back" calories. Is your choice worth the calories?

For the vegetables listed at right, visualize which category a vegetable might fit if not listed. For example: Is asparagus more like leafy greens and broccoli or more like corn? While asparagus is crunchy like both groups, there is no such thing as asparagus oil. Asparagus will fit the lower calorie group. Vegetables are so low in calories, you can't make a big mistake, even with starchy vegetables.

PRESCRIPTFIT®
MEDICAL NUTRITION THERAPY ▪ ▪ ▪ ▪ ▪ ▪ ▪

# CHAPTER 6: HEALING & EDUCATION

| VEGETABLE | CALORIES/ CUP* | AMOUNT OF VEGETABLE EQUIVALENT TO 1 BITE OF STEAK |
|---|---|---|
| Lettuce, Spinach, Turnip Greens, Cucumbers, Celery | 10 | 10 cups |
| Bell Pepper, Celery, Summer Squash (yellow) | 20 | 5 cups |
| Carrots, Asparagus, Okra, Green Beans, Cauliflower, Broccoli, Tomatoes | 40 | 3 cups |
| Onions | 60 | 2 cups |
| Eggplant, Cabbage, and Brussel Sprouts | 20 | 5 cups |

*These calorie contents are based on fresh preparation without condiments*

Though the vegetables listed below are a great caloric value compared to other food categories, they are higher in sugar and starch. Save these until Phase 13.

| VEGETABLE | CALORIES/ CUP* | AMT OF VEGETABLE EQUIVALENT TO 1 BITE OF STEAK |
|---|---|---|
| Winter Squash (Hubbard, Butternut, Acorn), Stewed Tomatoes | 80 | 1.5 cups |
| Fresh Peas. Fresh Beans, Diced Tomatoes | 120 | 1 cup |
| Corn, Mashed Potatoes | 140 | 1 cup |
| Dried Beans/Peas | 200 | 1 cup = 4 bites of steak or 2 miles of walking |

*These calorie contents are based on fresh preparation without condiments*

# SECTION B: DIVING IN...

### SHOPPING FOR VEGETABLES

Spend most of your grocery store time in the vegetable section, heading there right after seafood and poultry to reinforce Food Phase thinking. This is where you'll want to do the most planning since there are so many varieties and potential combinations that exist. Experiment with at least one new vegetable weekly. After shopping the fresh vegetable section, go directly to the canned or dried vegetable section to supplement your variety.

Look for condiments low in calories for dipping or mixing vegetables for salads. Avoid butter, cheese, and salad dressings with sugar or fat. Avoid any dressing over 20 calories/tablespoon. PrescriptFit salad dressing recipes contain less than 10 calories/tablespoon.

## MARY — GETTING KIDS TO EAT VEGETABLES

Mary is a loving mother whose kids sneer at vegetables and scream for pizza. Knowing the long-term health problems associated with poor nutrition, Mary developed a plan to change their eating habits.

First, she made the kids a deal that they could eat pizza twice a week if they had a PrescriptFit shake or pudding before and if they added one vegetable choice for every meat choice on their pizza.

Eventually she convinced the family to make pizza together, a fun activity that offered the bonus of making Mary more of a "culinary expert" in the household.

Two years later, Mary's kids are eating five cups of vegetables daily and paying a lot more attention to Mom's ideas on calories, nutrition, cooking, and what tastes "good."

Mary exhibited the patience and understanding necessary to change her family's eating habits. Habits and preferences are developed with practice. They take time, but are worth it!

**CASE STUDY**

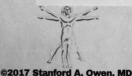

©2017 Stanford A. Owen, MD

# PRESCRIPTFIT®
MEDICAL NUTRITION THERAPY ▪ ▪ ▪ ▪ ▪ ▪ ▪

# CHAPTER 6: HEALING & EDUCATION

## COOKING & SEASONING VEGETABLES

A good way to eat your five servings of vegetables is to chop them and add to PrescriptFit Beef or Chicken soups. Broths are an excellent way to enhance vegetable flavor and variety without adding calories. Soups make excellent gravy when mixed thickly.

Baking or broiling vegetables also brings out vegetable flavor without soaking them in oil or butter. Chop up a variety of vegetables of different colors in about one-inch pieces. Place vegetables in a pan and spray with vegetable oil or butter spray (PAM™ has a nice selection). Broil the vegetables in the oven until slightly brown; sprinkling your favorite seasoning (ours is Paul Prudhomme's Magic Seasoning™ at www. chefpaul.com). Combining squash, asparagus, onion, bell pepper, and eggplant gets all the colors in a single, delicious dish.

*Raw vegetables are the most nutritious method of consuming vegetables. Leave raw vegetables displayed around the house and bring snack trays of vegetables and fruit to work.*

*Canned vegetables are equal in calories to fresh vegetables unless prepared with sugars or stew meats. Read the contents label on canned vegetables. They are mostly accurate.*

### BOB OWEN'S VEGETABLE RECIPES

- *Spinach & Artichoke Stuffed Tomato*
- *Onion Squash*
- *Lemon Broccoli*
- *Crispy Fresh Green Beans*
- *Hot Mustard Salad*
- *Salad Dressings*
  - *— Low-calorie Herb Vinaigrette*
  - *— Raspberry Vinaigrette*

*To access these and other great recipes, visit www.drdiet.com*
*Get started preparing tasty vegetable dishes.*

## PRESCRIPTFIT
MEDICAL NUTRITION THERAPY ▪ ▪ ▪ ▪ ▪ ▪ ▪

©2017 Stanford A. Owen, MD

# Section B: Diving In...

Reminder:

- Continue 6–8 or more PrescriptFit amino acid doses per day.

- Use PrescriptFit shakes or soups before or with meals.

- Use foods from Phases 2–8.

- Use Phase 13 foods for splurges ONLY.

- Take a multi-vitamin supplement.

- Drink 5 cups of water or calorie-free beverage daily.

National attention is now focused on disputing this myth. In December 2014, the U.S. government's Dietary Advisory Guidelines Committee reported that cholesterol is no longer considered a "nutrient of concern for overconsumption."

## Phase 5 Eggs

By now, if you've been following the PrescriptFit Plan, you are probably eager for each new Food Phase, for it adds to the variety of foods from which you can plan your meals.

### Eggs and Nutrition

Eggs are a wonderful addition to your meal planning for they are low in calories, filling, provide added taste and texture, and may be mixed with Food Phase 1–4 foods to create new recipes. Eggs do not cause dangerous insulin resistance or blood vessel malfunction. Eggs are high in protein and relatively low in fat, especially if the yolk is removed. However, egg yolk does contain a number of essential vitamins, and it is not necessary to always remove the yolk. Eggs are very inexpensive and can meet any budget. Eggs are for unlimited consumption. All you can eat!

### Egg Myths

The most stubborn myth about eggs is the concern that high cholesterol levels found in egg yolk will lead to atherosclerosis (cholesterol artery plaque). While the yolk does contain high amounts of cholesterol, cholesterol in food does not result in elevated blood cholesterol levels. Rather, sugar and saturated fat are the culprits that provoke the liver to manufacture and over-produce cholesterol.

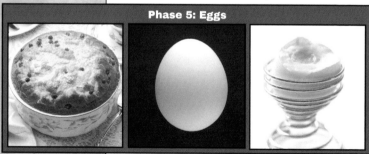

Phase 5: Eggs

**PRESCRIPTFIT**®
MEDICAL NUTRITION THERAPY ▪ ▪ ▪ ▪ ▪ ▪ ▪

# CHAPTER 6: HEALING & EDUCATION

Dietary cholesterol alone, when consumed without saturated fat or sugar, may actually decrease cholesterol production by the liver. For those skeptical about egg safety, simply limit egg consumption to three or fewer eggs per week. The true calorie danger in egg dishes comes with the addition of condiments. Avoid using cheese when preparing egg dishes. Cheese is composed mostly of saturated fat and is high calorie.

## CALORIES AND EGGS

Calories range between 80 and 90 calories per egg. For ease of remembering, just round it off to 100. One egg equals 100 calories, which would require one mile of walking for "payback." Egg yolk contains fat (at 9 calories/gram of fat). Egg white is pure protein (at 4 calories/gram). To cut back on calories, remove the yolk.

PrescriptFit Egg Pro™ product is pure egg-white powder. Egg Pro™ can be mixed with PrescriptFit shakes and soups or omelets to give more body and satiation.

> ### Dosing
>
> *No restriction — Enjoy eggs alone, in omelets with vegetables, or in mixed dishes based on what phase of the Plan you are currently following.*

*Egg white contains large amounts of the branched-chain amino acids that improve metabolism.*

## PEGGY — GETTING WELL & SAVING MONEY

I recently examined a 220-pound diabetic woman taking 20 different herbal and vitamin supplements per day, spending huge amounts of time on the Internet researching herb science, and feeling miserable with out-of-control diabetes and hypertension.

I discontinued all her herbs, saving her over $400 dollars per month, preventing unknown drug interactions, and simplifying her day immensely. She felt fantastic and gained perfect control of her diabetes and hypertension after only Food Phase 1 of the high risk (14-day) PrescriptFit MNT Plan, consuming only PrescriptFit amino acid shakes and soups and a single multiple vitamin.

She completed two sessions of the 13-Phase Plan and never needed medication again. She lost 80 pounds and returned to a full life. Her medication and herb bill dropped from $1,200/month to zero! I see similar cases every day in my clinic.

**CASE STUDY**

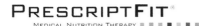

# PRESCRIPTFIT
MEDICAL NUTRITION THERAPY ▪ ▪ ▪ ▪ ▪ ▪ ▪

©2017 Stanford A. Owen, MD

# SECTION B: DIVING IN...

## Harold — A New Twist on the "Farm-Style" Breakfast

Harold came to our clinic to lose weight after suffering a heart attack. His cholesterol level was high; yet, he was essentially unaware of what cholesterol truly is and what can be done to control it. The only thing he was certain of was that cholesterol played a role in his heart attack, that the dietician at the hospital told him to avoid eggs, and that this was going to be a difficult change to make.

Having to give up the kind of breakfast he'd always known — sausage, eggs, biscuits, juice, whole milk — was very distressing for Harold. Moreover, his breakfast was a special time for him: a time of day spent with his wife (while the kids were still asleep).

I explained to Harold how current science has shown that the cytokine-provoking saturated fat in the sausage, biscuit, and whole milk was inflamed even further by the simple sugar in the biscuit and juice. It wasn't really the eggs that were the culprits in his "farm-style" breakfast; in fact, the cholesterol-like molecules in egg yolk might even be working to "turn off" cholesterol production by the liver.

Harold's wife came up with some creative substitutes — turkey sausage and a PrescriptFit shake for the pork sausage and whole milk and sugar-free Crystal Light™ instead of juice. She also eliminated the biscuit. Harold focused on cooking omelets and other egg dishes and became quite the chef. His cholesterol and weight dropped to normal ranges within six months without feeling deprived.

**CASE STUDY**

**PRESCRIPTFIT**®
MEDICAL NUTRITION THERAPY ■ ■ ■ ■ ■ ■ ■

# CHAPTER 6: HEALING & EDUCATION

## PHASE 6 NUTS

You may eat any variety of nuts on the PrescriptFit MNT Plan. All varieties are available year-round and each has its own unique flavor and texture. You can buy most nuts either shelled or unshelled. Unshelled nuts make great snacks, especially for the kids. Shell-cracking takes time (which limits caloric intake) and can be fun (or at least mesmerizing). Unshelled nuts may cost a little less.

Nuts are often considered snacks or party food, but they are especially useful as condiments on meat, vegetables, and dessert dishes.

Categories of nuts include: Walnuts, pecans, almonds, pistachios, peanuts, cashews, pine nuts, hickory nuts, chestnuts, acorns, Brazil nuts, and hazelnuts.

### NUTS AS NUTRITION

You may wonder why nuts, which are higher in fat, are added ahead of fruit in the Food Phase plan. There are several reasons:

> Nuts contain no carbohydrates and will not cause insulin resistance.

> Nut oils improve small blood vessel function, aiding in blood pressure and circulation.

### Dosing

*Nuts are one of the highest calorie/ounce foods at an average 175 calories per ounce. However, studies have demonstrated no weight gain in lean or obese individuals using nuts without restriction as a daily snack for six months. If you are susceptible to binge eating, you'll want to be extra careful with nuts. You should use primarily unshelled nuts or limit shelled nuts to no more than ¼ cup per day.*

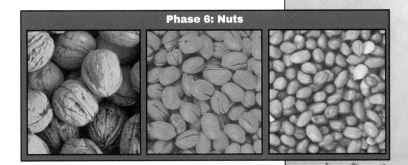

**Phase 6: Nuts**

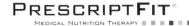

**PRESCRIPTFIT**®
MEDICAL NUTRITION THERAPY ▪ ▪ ▪ ▪ ▪ ▪ ▪

©2017 Stanford A. Owen, MD

# Section B: Diving In...

> The thin covering of certain nuts contain substances that lower cholesterol overall by raising "good" HDL cholesterol and lowering "bad" LDL cholesterol.

> While nuts are rich in oil (oil is 125 calories/tablespoon), one third of nut oil is not absorbed, instead passing through the intestine bound to nut fiber.

> Nuts are very satiating because nuts are high in protein and fat.

## Nut Myths

Salted nuts contain no more calories than unsalted nuts. However, you may need to avoid salted nuts if you have a medical condition that involves sensitivity to salt, such as congestive heart failure, kidney failure, and hypertension.

In addition to shelled or unshelled, salted or unsalted, you can also buy some nuts ground to use as a spread. Beware, however, that commercial peanut butter is often mixed with hydrogenated vegetable oil ("trans fat") to enhance texture, which ruins the health benefits of the nuts. If you have a health food store nearby, see if they have nut grinders for fresh nut spread.

**Taste tips:**

*The PrescriptFit Lactose-Free product whips into a thick pudding. The Lactose-Free product makes a nice dessert when mixed with chopped fruit, nuts, and spices.*

*Fresh peanut butter mixed (1 teaspoon) with PrescriptFit Chocolate (shake or pudding) is decadent!*

### BOB OWEN'S NUT RECIPES

- *Toasted Almonds*
- *Candied Pecans*
- *Salted Walnuts*

*To access these and other great recipes, view the Recipe section at www.drdiet.com*

*Get started preparing tasty nut dishes.*

**PRESCRIPTFIT**®
MEDICAL NUTRITION THERAPY ▪ ▪ ▪ ▪ ▪ ▪

# ～ CHAPTER 6: HEALING & EDUCATION ～

## PHASE 7 FRUIT

Some of you who love fruit are now saying, "Ah, at last I can add fruit to my meal plan!" Others of you may have learned to fear fruit for its carbohydrate content. Fruit should not be feared, but it is added in the second half of the PrescriptFit MNT Plan since fruit is primarily carbohydrate. If you have a medical condition sensitive to sugar, you'll want to ask your health care provider to monitor your condition closely during Food Phase 7.

## FRUIT AS NUTRITION

Fresh fruit contains carbohydrate and fiber as primary nutrients; some fruits contain small amounts of fat (avocado). Fruits also contain vitamins and minerals, especially vitamin C, and minimal amounts of protein.

Although you can get the same vitamins and minerals in pills with zero calories and the same amount of fiber from food supplement powders, natural fruit has its advantages. For one thing, it has "entertainment" value because it tastes good. Unlike other entertainment foods that contain processed sugars, the sugar in fruit is contained and inter-twined with the fiber, causing a slow release of sugar into the bloodstream — known as "glycemic index." The more rapidly sugar enters the bloodstream, the higher the glycemic index.

### Dosing

*If fruit is raw or whole, "overdose" on fruit calories is very unlikely. Therefore, the PrescriptFit MNT Plan does not restrict fruit consumption.*

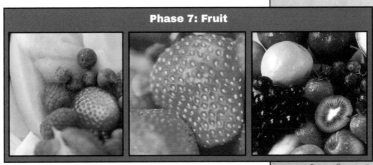

**Phase 7: Fruit**

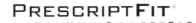

# PRESCRIPTFIT

MEDICAL NUTRITION THERAPY ▪ ▪ ▪ ▪ ▪ ▪ ▪

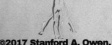

# SECTION B: DIVING IN...

All fruit has a relatively low glycemic index compared to "high glycemic index" soft drinks, juices, and snacks. Fruit can satisfy your "sweet tooth" without the huge doses of sugar from refined products. How many pieces of fruit would it take to squeeze one glass of orange, grapefruit, grape, pineapple, apple, or other juices? Imagine eating that many pieces of fruit in the 30 seconds it takes you to gulp down a glass of juice or soda! If you replace one refined snack or glass of juice with a piece of fresh fruit, the benefit is huge.

## CATEGORIES OF FRUIT

There are too many categories or varieties of fruit to name here. Challenge yourself and your family to try new fruits along with the familiar and customary varieties you may already eat regularly. If you are already accustomed to eating oranges, apples, bananas, grapes, strawberries, or melon, try kiwi or blueberries. Remember to experiment with a variety of colors. As you try new varieties of fruit, ask each member of the family for their opinion. Kids, in particular, are open to new tastes if challenged with variety early in life. Don't make a big deal about the "new" fruit. Instead be a role model for your family, willing to try new tastes, and express your reaction with adjectives like "yummy" or "phenomenal."

## CALORIES IN FRUIT

Fruit calories are measured in ounces, from 5 calories per ounce (lemon and tomato) to 45 calories per ounce (avocado). These are very low calories per ounce compared to almost any other food choice. Even avocado, at 45 calories per ounce, is less than chicken (50 calories per ounce). The reason fruit is placed in Food Phase 7, rather than an earlier Food Phase, is that fruit is not very satiating. Fruit does not "fill" or "stick

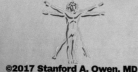

PRESCRIPTFIT®
MEDICAL NUTRITION THERAPY ■ ■ ■ ■ ■ ■ ■

# ∼ Chapter 6: Healing & Education ∼

to the ribs," so eating fruit will not usually reduce overall calorie intake; you'll still feel hungry for something else. Fruit is very tasty and should be considered a "treat" for the sweet tooth.

Thousands of fruit varieties from all parts of the world are now available in our local stores. If a particular fruit is not listed below, guess which type it would be most similar to.

*Fruit is low in calories per ounce. Use the chart below to compare the caloric content of your favorite fruits. If a particular fruit is not listed, ask yourself if it is more like one of those listed below.*

| Fruit | Calories/ Ounce | Amount = to about 100 calories or burned in walking one mile |
|---|---|---|
| Lemon, Tomato | 5 | 20 ounces |
| Melons | 10 | ¼ watermelon |
| Apple, Pineapple, Orange | 15 | 2 |
| Grapes | 20 | 1 large bowl |
| Banana | 30 | 1 banana |
| Avocado | 45 | About ½ avocado |
| Dried fruit | 85 | **Avoid as is very calorie-dense when limiting calories** |

It is more important to enjoy a particular fruit than "sweat" the calories. If you and your family enjoy a fruit, you are more likely to consume them daily and forego less nutritious snacks.

Keep fruit in front of your face from Food Phase 7 forward. Replace refined sugar snacks with fruit, nuts, or PrescriptFit snack bars. Place them on the counter, in the den, and around the television or computer.

Buy and mix as many colors and varieties as possible. Each color represents different nutrients and vitamins, different tastes, and additional options for the picky eaters in your family.

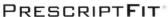

PRESCRIPTFIT
MEDICAL NUTRITION THERAPY ▪ ▪ ▪ ▪ ▪ ▪ ▪

# Section B: Diving In...

## PHASE 8: SNACKS

Snacks are a part of modern Western culture. For some people snacks are so handy and tempting they lead to unconscious over-consumption. The solution is usually not to deprive ourselves of snacks but to learn to choose snacks that are healthy alternatives.

All PrescriptFit snacks are high in protein, low in glycemic sugars (sucrose), and they taste good! You'll probably find that you can replace your typical household snacks for kids and spouses with PrescriptFit snack bars and crisps. If you're doubtful, don't tell them that you are using "diet food," and see if they notice the difference. More than likely, they'll demand you keep these items around, making your diet tasks easier.

In addition to PrescriptFit snacks, you can always use fruits and nuts as healthy snack alternatives.

Most PrescriptFit snacks are made from nonfat dry milk, egg white, soy proteins, and artificial sweeteners. The chocolate snack is made from the highest quality cocoa, an excellent antioxidant

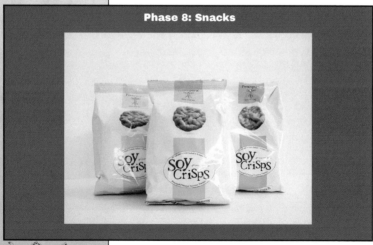

**Phase 8: Snacks**

©2017 Stanford A. Owen, MD

**PRESCRIPTFIT®**
MEDICAL NUTRITION THERAPY ▪ ▪ ▪ ▪ ▪ ▪ ▪

that has direct beneficial effects on small blood vessels. You may also use these products as a dessert or as a meal replacement. A shake and snack bar is a filling meal. Unless consumed in large quantities, snack bars should not induce cytokine production from fat cells.

PrescriptFit bars taste as good as candy bars, but they are far different. Commercial candy bars are made with sucrose (sugar) and large amounts of hydrogenated vegetable oils. They are huge, with 3–4 times the calories as PrescriptFit snack bars.

If chips and pastries are your weakness, consider this: All varieties have about 125 calories per ounce. And if you are one who "can't eat just one," those calories will add up quickly, along with the fat. You'll be much more successful at achieving and maintaining your desired weight and fitness level if you ban the chips and pastries and choose fruit, nuts, or PrescriptFit bars and soy crisps instead.

### Dosing

Unlimited. For an extra treat, crumble PrescriptFit bar over a PrescriptFit pudding.

## PRESCRIPTFIT SNACK BARS

All PrescriptFit Snack Bars average about 150 calories. All are high protein (about 50 percent), very satiating, and they taste great.

The bars can be used as a snack or meal replacement. Protein content is soy, egg white, and milk solids. A snack bar and shake is great choice for lunch, after school snack, or for dessert!

Try these bar flavors:

- Cinnamon Crunch
- Peanut Crunch
- Coconut
- Double Berry
- Sweet & Salty
- Chocolate
- Toffee

- Lemon Meringue
- Butter Pecan
- Brownie
- Peanut Butter Crunch
- Almond
- Fudge Graham
- Chocolate Mint

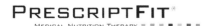

PRESCRIPTFIT
MEDICAL NUTRITION THERAPY ▪ ▪ ▪ ▪ ▪ ▪ ▪

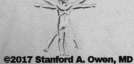

©2017 Stanford A. Owen, MD

# SECTION B: DIVING IN...

## Splurging and PrescriptFit

The "splurge" meal concept was developed after polling patients in our clinic about how many high-calorie, high-fat, "fun" (as described by those polled) meals are absolutely essential for quality life. From this poll, we reached two overwhelming conclusions:

1. Ninety percent of those polled stated that five to ten meals per month were "essential." Their comments frequently sounded like this, "I live in the New Orleans area, where food is a crucial ingredient of our way of life. It is as essential as the music to our festivities and culture as a whole."

   In New Orleans, eating is entertainment. Yet, most New Orleaneans agree that two to three meals per week at a world-class eatery is adequate (even if price is not an issue). Give this some thought, and ask your spouse or friends. Most will agree.

2. Participants who recorded splurge meals for the coming month had something of an "epiphany." When actually writing down all the unexpected but planned events that resulted in "splurging," people could easily see what accounted for the many pounds gained in a given year.

All participants of the poll used the PrescriptFit Calendar. If you can't seem to determine where those extra pounds came from, use the PrescriptFit™ Calendar — it works!

**CASE STUDY**

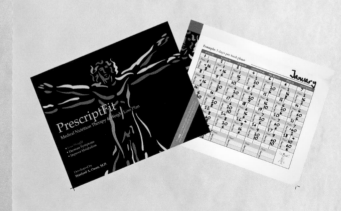

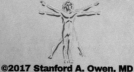

©2017 Stanford A. Owen, MD

# PRESCRIPTFIT®
MEDICAL NUTRITION THERAPY ▪ ▪ ▪ ▪ ▪ ▪ ▪

# CHAPTER 7: SPLURGING

## CHAPTER 7: LET'S SPLURGE! — PHASES 9–13

### SPECIAL MEALS FOR SPECIAL OCCASIONS

**Merriam-Webster Dictionary** defines the verb, "to splurge," as "To indulge oneself extravagantly." Whether we are being extravagant with our money, say, indulging in a new outfit, or extravagant with our food choices, it is not something we do every day. If we did, we wouldn't get that special thrill we feel when we break through our normal restraints and behave extravagantly!

In the context of PrescriptFit MNT, we use "splurging" to describe a special meal, usually involving entertainment or social interaction. Generally, most meals used for such purposes are higher in fat, carbohydrate, and calories than the routine meals that have become our norm on the Food Phase Plan.

Most restaurant meals would be considered "splurge" meals. Most family feasts are splurge meals. Some business meetings might qualify as splurge meals. Many vacation meals would be splurge meals. Life crises definitely throw unplanned meals your way. I call "splurge" meals my "Weekends, Weddings, and Wakes" solution.

Alcoholic beverages are also considered "splurge" items. Alcohol is usually consumed in high-calorie environments and will lower inhibitions in anyone attempting food avoidance — so why try? Go with it. Add the alcohol to the "splurge" and pay back later.

Medical Treatment

PrescriptFit®

Splurging

Healing & Education

**PRESCRIPTFIT**
MEDICAL NUTRITION THERAPY

# Section B: Diving In...

Eight splurge meals are allowed every month.

"Splurge" meals should be enjoyed. Do not restrict portions. Do not strain your brain. Try to plan "splurge" meals through the month by placing them on your PrescriptFit Calendar at the beginning of the month. BUT if a "splurge" opportunity comes your way unplanned, enjoy the event. Simply replace a previously planned "splurge" meal on the Calendar the following day. For many, this will be an eye-opening experience. It may take practice and patience to hold total "splurge" meals to eight or less per month.

Splurging also allows for extended diet distractions such as a vacation or life crises. All eight splurge meals may be used consecutively, such as an extended trip or vacation. When (not if) crises hit, the splurge meals can also be counted consecutively until you're through the crisis. Simply replace future splurge meals until they are balanced out. This may take several months. No big deal!

Splurging is a unique concept of the Plan. The simple fact is eight meals per month out of a potential ninety meal slots (3 meals per day times 30 days per month) is not going to make someone obese or drastically alter their disease stability.

Splurging allows you to integrate your real life with your structured diet plan. It works!

Accountability is a vital component of any successful diet method. Many diet plans require weekly meetings to enforce accountability. With PrescriptFit MNT, you hold yourself accountable by using the PrescriptFit Calendar. (See pages 42–43 for complete directions on using the Calendar.)

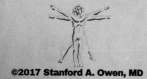

**PRESCRIPTFIT**
MEDICAL NUTRITION THERAPY ▪ ▪ ▪ ▪ ▪ ▪ ▪

# ⌐ CHAPTER 7: SPLURGING ⌐

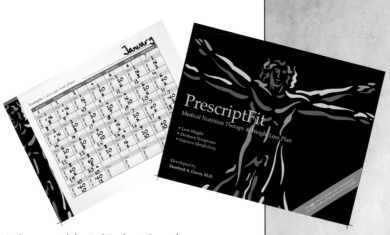

Mark your anticipated "splurge" meals on your Calendar at the beginning of the month. When you have unanticipated splurging, mark those meals on the calendar and remove a planned splurge meal. If you update your Calendar daily, you will be accountable daily, not weekly, for your success or failure. Demonstrate accountability to your healthcare provider by bringing your disease/symptom questionnaires (from section C) to your medical appointments.

Role model accountability for your family and friends by sharing your strategies and results. You never know how you might help others improve their own health by being a positive example.

*If real people are going to follow a diet plan forever, the diet plan has to function in the real world. Splurging and feasting are as old as civilization. Our entire culture is built around feasting, family, and friends. Any diet that does not consider this fact will fail.*

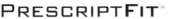

# PRESCRIPTFIT®
MEDICAL NUTRITION THERAPY ■ ■ ■ ■ ■ ■ ■

# SECTION B: DIVING IN...

## PHASE 9 PORK

Promoters call pork, "the other white meat," referring to poultry or fish. However, pork is not poultry or fish. Even the leanest cuts of pork have substantial saturated fat and calories. Pork is pork and should not be substituted for poultry or fish as a major component of your diet.

### PORK AS NUTRITION

Pork and beef could be considered nutritionally comparable. They are placed in separate Food Phases primarily to encourage skill training with recipes. Pork varies in fat content with cut and individual carcass fat. Pork from wild hogs is quite lean, approaching fat content in poultry. Commercially raised pork averages 100–125 calories per ounce.

Pork contains no carbohydrate. The leanest pork cut (pork loin) averages about 100 calories/ounce. You can trim some of the calories by trimming away any visible excess fat. However, most fat is mingled or "marbleized" into pork meat and cannot be easily removed with trimming.

Pork fat is saturated fat that induces the liver to manufacture excessive cholesterol, especially the "bad" or harmful LDL cholesterol particles that inflame arteries. Saturated fat induces insulin malfunction or "resistance," increases cytokine production, and

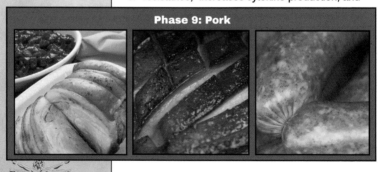

**Phase 9: Pork**

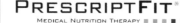

# ⟿ CHAPTER 7: SPLURGING ⟿

impairs small blood vessel function, leading to hypertension and fluid retention.

Some individuals are more sensitive to the adverse effects of saturated fat than others. Those with heart attack or stroke in the family, elevated cholesterol levels, diabetes, or pre-diabetes (IRS), should be especially careful when adding the pork Food Phase to the Plan. If you have diabetes, pre-diabetes, or heart disease, work with your health care provider to monitor blood pressure, sudden increase in scale weight (fluid retention), blood sugar, cholesterol, and triglycerides.

## CATEGORIES OF PORK AND CALORIES

Pork is made from hogs; preparation of the meat results in different fat or calorie content.

> Ham (smoked pork treated with sugar)

> Sausage (ground pork, usually with added fat)

> Deli meats (processed pork)

> Chops and roasts

Pork averages between 100 and 125 calories per ounce, with pork loin on the lean end and pork chops on the fatter end of pork cuts. Sausage tops out at about 150 calories/ounce (about the same as heavy pies or cheesecake).

## SPLURGING WITH PORK

Mark your PrescriptFit Calendar at the beginning of each month and mark off eight allowed "splurge" meals. Use a splurge meal for pork, beef, dairy, or baked foods; where you can:

> Eat as much of the splurge item(s) as desired but only for that meal.

> Mix pork with foods from Food Phases 1–8 to achieve calorie balance and to limit "damage" from that splurge meal.

---

### Dosing

**Splurge Only! Because pork is high in calories and harmful saturated fat, it should be consumed at "splurge" meals, no more than eight per month.**

### BOB OWEN'S PORK RECIPES

- **Smothered Pork Tenderloin**
- **Asian Pork**
- **Barbecued Pork Loin**
- **Rosemary Roasted Pork Tenderloin**

*To access these and other great recipes, visit www.drdiet.com*

*Get started preparing tasty pork dishes.*

---

## PRESCRIPTFIT®

MEDICAL NUTRITION THERAPY ▪ ▪ ▪ ▪ ▪ ▪ ▪ ▪

# Section B: Diving In...

*Combine beef with other foods for healthier splurge meals. "Medley" recipes, such as Shish Kabob, are a great way to fill up on vegetables while keeping beef volume down. Be sure to mark your eight "splurge" meals on your PrescriptFit Calendar.*

## Phase 10 Beef

Beef is easily America's favorite food. But because beef is loaded with harmful saturated fat and calories, and is easily consumed to excess, consider it a "splurge" item for your monthly food calendar.

### Beef as Nutrition

Beef contains no carbohydrates and is composed mainly of protein and fat. The fat is "marbleized" into the meat. If you "fry" beef, little extra fat enters the meat since it is already saturated. To minimize calories, trim excess fat from the meat prior to cooking.

Lean cuts of beef (round roasts or steak, chuck) have approximately 100 calories per ounce while heavier cuts of beef (sirloin, rib-eye, T-bone) average about 125 calories per ounce. Cooking the fat out of the meat is helpful to reduce the calories, but why bother? If you are going to use beef as a "treat" (eight splurge meals per month), why remove the substance that provides the "treat" — the fat?

### Categories of Beef and Calories

Most people are familiar with beef cuts and marbleized fat in beef. When cattle are fed regular feed and have moderate marbleized fat, they

**Phase 10: Beef**

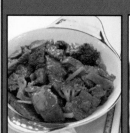
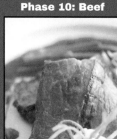
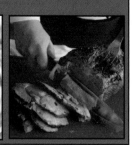

## PRESCRIPTFIT®
MEDICAL NUTRITION THERAPY

# ⁓ CHAPTER 7: SPLURGING ⁓

produce "choice" cuts of beef. Those fed high grades of feed, usually corn, have more marbleized fat, producing "prime" cuts. Most people think prime cuts taste better since they contain more fat.

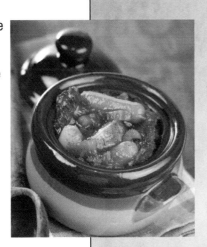

Highest fat cuts include:

> Rib-eye
> Sirloin
> T-bone
> Strip (sirloin)
> Porterhouse
> Tenderloin (Filet Mignon)

Leaner cuts include round steak, roasts, and chuck. Ground beef is mixed with "parts" of other beef, usually fat scraps, used as fillers. Ground beef marked as "95 percent fat free" is very inaccurate.

All beef is at least 50 percent fat; therefore, "percent fat" is a marketing gimmick that ends up falsely assuring you the product is not harmful to your health.

## Randy — The Beef Guy

Randy is a serious, barbecue guy. He tailgates every chance he gets and invites friends over for BBQ most every weekend. Randy never misses a BBQ episode on the *Food Network*.

Even Randy was surprised that "splurging" on BBQ beef, pork, or chicken was more than adequate two days each week. He was quite satisfied to grill seafood, poultry, and vegetables the remaining days.

He was so taken with the diet plan he "took over" cooking two meals normally prepared each week by his wife. Randy's wife is very happy with PrescriptFit!

**CASE STUDY**

# PRESCRIPTFIT®
MEDICAL NUTRITION THERAPY ▪ ▪ ▪ ▪ ▪ ▪ ▪

# SECTION B: DIVING IN...

Here's something to think about: If fish and beef contain no carbohydrate, why does beef contain 125 calories per ounce and fish only 25 calories per ounce? Fat! Remember: fat contains 9 calories per gram while protein and carbohydrate contain 4 calories per gram.

## BOB OWEN'S BEEF RECIPES

- **Smothered Round Steak**
- **Sweet & Spicy Beef (may substitute chicken or pork)**
- **Skillet Steak in Wild Mushroom & Roasted Garlic Sauce**
- **Beef and Vegetable Stew**

*To access these and other great recipes, visit www.drdiet.com*

*Get started preparing tasty beef dishes.*

## GINGER — MANAGING LIQUID CALORIES

Ginger and her coworkers enjoyed meeting after work at the pub just around the corner from office. Being single, Ginger tended to join the group two or three evenings a week rather than going home to an empty apartment.

A problem Ginger didn't count on (literally) involved the calories she consumed sharing pitchers of beer (plus the occasional high-fat appetizer plate) on such a frequent basis. Ginger had gained 40 pounds in the past year. She attributed her more frequent drinking with her friends to needing to relieve some of the "stress" at work and to being lonely.

I suggested Ginger save the drinking for "TGIFs" once her weight was back under control. I strongly recommended she exchange the time at the pub for time at the gym, perhaps getting some of her friends to join with her. Exercise helps with mental health as much as physical health. Moreover, exercise has been shown to significantly decrease the "stress" Ginger complained of from her job.

Ginger met Buddy later that year at the gym. She is now married, and has a baby boy. She feels and looks great and finds TGIF more than adequate to quench her partying soul and stay connected with her friends.

**CASE STUDY**

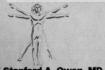

# CHAPTER 7: SPLURGING

## PHASE 11 BEVERAGES

We recommend you save your beverages for your eight splurge meals (events) per month. For example, PrescriptFit shakes mixed with alcoholic beverages can help you limit your calorie consumption because the drinks are filling while supplying some of your amino acid daily dose recommendations.

## BEVERAGES AS NUTRITION

Elimination of caloric (calorie containing) beverages is the single most substantial act you can take to minimize calories with any diet. We often consume beverages hurriedly and without much sensation of fullness or satiation. Seldom do we finish a beverage and say, "Wow, what a memorable experience." Therefore, caloric beverages are truly "empty" calories — empty nutrition and empty pleasure. Any and all diet (zero calorie) beverages are allowed with the Plan.

Milk is the only caloric beverage of sufficient nutrient value to consider using as a nutritious beverage. However, whole milk contains over 50 percent saturated fat by dry weight; 2 percent milk is about 35 percent saturated fat by dry weight; skim milk contains about 10 percent saturated fat. Only powdered nonfat milk is completely devoid of dangerous saturated fat. Most people

### Dosing

*Splurge Only! Because beverages are high in calories, they should be consumed at "splurge" meals, no more than eight per month.*

*The Centers for Disease Control notes the #1 cause of preventable cancer is not cigarettes, but obesity. The #1 contributor to obesity is consuming caloric beverages.*

**Phase 11: Beverages**

## PRESCRIPTFIT
MEDICAL NUTRITION THERAPY ■ ■ ■ ■ ■ ■ ■

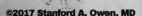

©2017 Stanford A. Owen, MD

# SECTION B: DIVING IN...

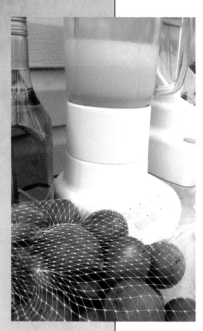

are not willing to put up with the taste of powdered nonfat milk for routine consumption. Milk tastes good because of the saturated fat. Saturated fat is "sticky." It sticks to your arteries like milk sticks to your lip or butter to your hand. Saturated fat has adverse effects on blood vessel and insulin function. Therefore, if milk must be consumed, skim or nonfat milk are the best options.

Nonfat milk contains protein and complex carbohydrates. It also contains substantial amounts of calcium. Dietary calcium has been associated with weight loss and health benefits. Calcium directly suppresses cytokine production in fat cells and the liver. PrescriptFit amino acid shakes and soups contain nonfat milk solids with 100 percent of adult daily calcium requirements. No extra calcium supplements are needed with five or more PrescriptFit doses per day.

Alcoholic beverages have demonstrated protection against heart attack and stroke. However, what dose of alcohol provides best protection is unclear. Due to calorie considerations and toxic effects of high alcohol doses, alcoholic beverages are placed in the "splurge" meal categories — eight meals (events) per month.

## BEVERAGE MYTHS

The notion that juice is a "healthy" beverage is badly misplaced. Concentrated sugar is not healthy in any form — including juices. Many juices have added sugar or have been concentrated to increase sweetness. Juices fortified with calcium

### Reminder:

- Continue 6–8 or more PrescriptFit amino acid doses per day.

- Use PrescriptFit shakes or soups before or with meals.

- Use foods from Phases 2–8.

- Use Phase 13 foods for splurges ONLY.

- Take a multi-vitamin supplement.

- Drink 5 cups of water or calorie-free beverage daily.

PRESCRIPTFIT
MEDICAL NUTRITION THERAPY ▪ ▪ ▪ ▪ ▪ ▪ ▪

# �býⲤⲎⲀⲢⲦⲈⲢ 7: SⲢⳑⲨⲢⲄⲒⲚⲄ ⟩

or vitamins have far less calcium or vitamins than can be obtained from a non-caloric vitamin or mineral supplement.

Milk has been promoted as nature's most "perfect food." It is — if you're an infant animal with a growing nervous system that needs fat for growth. However, the saturated fat in milk is harmful to adult arteries.

Sports drinks contain sugar and calories, and they contribute to obesity and insulin resistance. Avoid sports drinks.

The worst myth is "diet" drinks that contain saccharin or aspartame are harmful. Data about harm are virtually non-existent while safety data on these products are abundant. Compared to sugar in soft drinks, artificial sweeteners are infinitely less harmful. On pages 36-40, you will find an in-depth treatment of sweeteners — artificial and natural that explains the impact of ingesting sugar with liquids. Also in that section, you will find a discussion of how the research supports the safety of artificial sweeteners.

When you compare beverages in the chart below, remember that it takes one mile of walking to burn 100 calories!

**BOB OWEN'S PRESCRIPTFIT BEVERAGE RECIPES**

- Pina Colada
- Strawberry Daiquiri
- Banana Banshee
- Tropical Fruit Delight
- Calypso Fudge
- Cappuccino Kahlua® Delight
- Mango Daiquiri
- Crème de Lite

To access these PrescriptFit beverage recipes, visit www.drdiet.com

| BEVERAGE | CALORIES/ OUNCE | WALKING DISTANCE REQUIRED TO BURN THOSE CALORIES |
|----------|-----------------|--------------------------------------------------|
| Diet drinks | 0 | 0 |
| Soft drinks | 12 | 1.5 miles per 12-ounce can |
| Beer | 12 | 1.5 miles per 12-ounce can |
| Juice | 20 | 1.5 miles per 8-ounce glass |
| Milk | 20 | 1.5 miles per 8-ounce glass |
| Wine | 20 | 1 mile per 4- to 6-ounce glass |
| Liquor | 60 | 1 mile per 1 ½-ounce shot |
| Liqueur | 100–150 | 2 miles per shot |

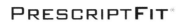

PRESCRIPTFIT®
MEDICAL NUTRITION THERAPY ▪ ▪ ▪ ▪ ▪ ▪ ▪

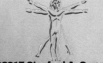

©2017 Stanford A. Owen, MD

# Section B: Diving In...

The three main sources of harmful saturated fat in modern diets are:

- Fried Foods
- Dairy Products
- Fatty meats

## Phase 12 Dairy

Dairy is added in the final PrescriptFit Phases since dairy products are easy to over-consume. Dairy can be harmful or healthful, depending on the type and amount consumed.

### Dairy Categories

- > Milk
- > Buttermilk
- > Cream
- > Cheese
- > Cottage cheese
- > Yogurt
- > Ice cream
- > Sour cream
- > Cream cheese
- > Whipped creams

### Dairy Nutrition

Most dairy products are now available in nonfat varieties. Dairy products that would traditionally contain sugar, like ice cream, can be made with artificial sweeteners and nonfat milk, decreasing fat and calories. Dairy should be considered a condiment to enhance flavors in Food Phases 1–11 or as a stand-alone treat for dessert.

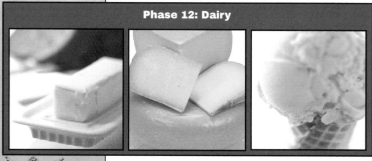

Phase 12: Dairy

**PRESCRIPTFIT**®
MEDICAL NUTRITION THERAPY ▪ ▪ ▪ ▪ ▪ ▪ ▪

# CHAPTER 7: SPLURGING

Dairy products made from whole milk contain about 50 percent of calories from fat, 30 percent from carbohydrate, and 20 percent from protein. The fat is harmful saturated fat. Nonfat milk contains about 60 percent complex carbohydrate and 40 percent protein (whey).

## DAIRY MYTHS

We've all grown up believing the myth that milk is essential for growth and development after infancy. However, we are the only species that consumes milk after infancy. Certainly calcium is beneficial for bone density, especially during the growth spurt in adolescent children. But calcium is readily available from many sources of less-fattening foods, such as vegetables.

The PrescriptFit product dosing is designed to provide enough calcium to the daily diet without the need for extra calcium supplementation — about 1,500 mg/day.

Clearly those items with the most fat have the most calories. Those with the most calories are also most harmful to arteries and abnormal metabolism.

### Reminder:

- Continue 6–8 or more PrescriptFit amino acid doses per day.

- Use PrescriptFit shakes or soups before or with meals.

- Use foods from Phases 2–8.

- Use Phase 13 foods for splurges ONLY.

- Take a multi-vitamin supplement.

- Drink 5 cups of water or calorie-free beverage daily.

## Wilson — Victim of Dairy Overload

Wilson weighed 550 pounds when he came to our clinic, claiming he didn't eat "anything." On interview, I found he didn't "eat anything" indeed. He drank everything — two gallons of whole milk per day and a liter of cola — that's about 6,000 calories per day of milk alone. I calculated he should weigh even more!

Marketed as a "health food" for over 50 years, dairy is a major culprit in the epidemic of obesity. One glass of milk at 150 calories, seven days per week, four weeks per month, and 52 weeks per year equals 54,750 calories or 16 pounds per year. Worth it? Maybe.

Perhaps those 54,750 calories would be better enjoyed on a Splurge?

**CASE STUDY**

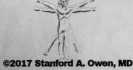

# SECTION B: DIVING IN...

### DAIRY DOSING ADVICE

*Nonfat cheese is equivalent to seafood or poultry and may be used as replacement for those choices. Use regular cheese only for splurge meals.*

Only nonfat cottage cheese, nonfat cheese, and nonfat yogurt are allowed in unlimited doses since their calorie content is equivalent to seafood. They may even be used in place of seafood or poultry as a main dish or "entrée" meal component. Nonfat sour cream and cream cheese should be used sparingly as a condiment. Ice cream and cream dishes should be used only on "splurge" meals. The chart on the next page outlines specific dosing advice.

How far would you need to walk in a month to pay back one glass of milk per day? A whopping 44 miles! Avoid milk.

| DAIRY FOOD | CALORIES PER OUNCE | CALORIES PER TYPICAL SERVING |
|---|---|---|
| Yogurt (regular) | 50 | 200 |
| Yogurt (nonfat) | 25 | 100 |
| Sour cream (regular) | 50 | 200 |
| Sour cream (nonfat) | 30 | 100 |
| Cream cheese (regular) | 75 | 200 |
| Cream cheese (nonfat) | 30 | 100 |
| Cheese (regular) | 100 | 400 |
| Cheese (nonfat) | 25 | 200 |
| Ice cream (regular) | 125–150 | 500–1000 |
| Milk | 20 | 160 |
| Cream | 75 | 400 |

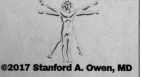

**PRESCRIPTFIT**®
MEDICAL NUTRITION THERAPY ▪ ▪ ▪ ▪ ▪ ▪ ▪ ▪

# ⇒ CHAPTER 7: SPLURGING ⇒

## DAIRY DOSING ADVICE

| Cottage Cheese (nonfat) | Yogurt |
|---|---|
| Use in place of seafood or poultry for a "meat" selection (but not until after you have reached Food Phase 12 in sequence). Nonfat cottage cheese is almost pure protein at 25 calories per ounce. You can mix it with fresh or canned fruit for flavor or use Splenda™ if you want a "sweet" taste. As with fish and poultry, you can eat unlimited amounts of nonfat cottage cheese. | Yogurt, preferably nonfat or low-fat yogurt, may be used as a main serving or a dessert. It is especially tasty as a dessert with fresh fruit or mixed with nuts. Be sure to measure your serving size carefully because it's easy to over-consume yogurt. You'll need to walk a couple of miles to pay back the calories in a typical carton of yogurt; less if it is nonfat yogurt. |
| **Sour Cream and Cream Cheese** | **Cream, Cheese, and Ice Cream (Splurge ONLY)** |
| These two condiments should be used on vegetables and selected meat dishes. Nonfat varieties are available; however, careful dosing is suggested. | Use these items only for your eight "splurge" meals per month. At 100-150 calories per ounce, they have the same caloric content and saturated fat as beef or pork. They can cause serious harm to those with diabetes, hypertension, and heart disease. |
| **Cheese (nonfat)** | **Whipped Cream (nonfat)** |
| Nonfat cheese is equivalent to seafood or poultry and may be used as replacement for those choices. | You may use unlimited amounts of the nonfat variety on desserts, puddings, nuts, etc. Avoid the full-fat version. |

## Milk, Buttermilk, Cream

Avoid these dairy products due to the tendency to over consume excess calories and fat.

### BOB OWEN'S DAIRY RECIPES

- Lemon Yogurt
- Squash Soup
- Jalapeño Cream Cheese Dip
- Chocolate Cream Pie

*To access these and other great recipes, visit www.drdiet.com*

*Get started preparing these and other great dairy recipes.*

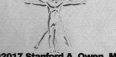

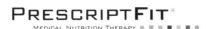

## PRESCRIPTFIT®
MEDICAL NUTRITION THERAPY ▪ ▪ ▪ ▪ ▪ ▪ ▪     ©2017 Stanford A. Owen, MD

# Section B: Diving In...

*Consider this:*

*Muffins sold at airport
deli stands average
10-12 ounces per
muffin (or 1,000
calories!).*

*A large piece of pecan
pie will require up to
10 miles of walking
payback!*

## Phase 13 Starches

Starches are simple carbohydrates found in wheat, corn, rice, and potatoes. They are also found in legumes but are less in percentage (with protein) and bound to fiber more tightly, preventing rapid absorption.

Refined carbohydrates are created when wheat, corn, rice, and potatoes are crushed, usually into powder. This makes the sugars available for your body to rapidly absorb them through the intestinal wall into your bloodstream. Once these sugars flood your bloodstream, they stress the insulin-producing pancreas and provoke a flood of toxic cytokines from fat, liver, and intestine. This insulin-cytokine response is especially intense when you eat foods that combine fat and starch, such as cereal and milk, bread and butter, pasta and cream sauce, rice and gravy, potatoes and sour cream, or fried potatoes. Other examples of combining a fat plus sugars (carbs) include chips, snacks, cake, and cookies.

The intestinal and fat-produced cytokines provoked by these fat-carb combinations are especially stimulating to the brain, making these foods irresistible or addicting, especially for those with type 2 diabetes. The reason we reserve starches for Phase 13 is to allow the addicted,

**Phase 13: Starches**

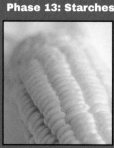
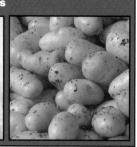

**PrescriptFit**®
MEDICAL NUTRITION THERAPY ▪ ▪ ▪ ▪ ▪ ▪ ▪

# CHAPTER 7: SPLURGING

carb-conditioned brain to "detox," decreasing the powerful allure of these foods. Once "detoxed," many patients find they are able to face these foods with more control, such as the twice per week Splurge strategy used with PrescriptFit MNT.

## STARCHY FOODS AND NUTRITION

Starchy foods — including starchy vegetables and baked goods — are reserved for the final Phase of the Plan because these foods are most likely to induce symptoms and weight gain. The reasons are clear:

> Baked goods are higher in calories per ounce compared to foods in Food Phases 1–8.

> Baked goods contain refined carbohydrates and fat (usually saturated or "trans" vegetable fat) that is quickly absorbed — the so-called "glycemic" effect that promotes insulin release, insulin resistance, and cytokine production.

> Baked goods are very tasty because of the sugar-fat combination, and are easily over consumed. Yet they are not filling, leading to even more consumption.

> Starchy vegetables are considerably lower in calories and fat than most baked goods, but can be over-consumed.

## STARCH TRUTHS AND MYTHS

"Carb" has become a four-letter word. Even more trendy, "gluten" bashing is all the rage. Are carbs and "gluten" really that harmful?

My experience is that patients feel dramatically better when avoiding the combination of fat and starches. They feel dramatically and rapidly worse, even after one meal, when binging on the fat-carb combination. The simplistic explanation of "gluten"

---

*The caloric content of most baked goods is as high or higher than beef or pork, is far less satiating or filling, and will contribute to:*

- *Excess insulin secretion*
- *Insulin resistance*
- *Excess cytokine production*

---

### Reminder:

- *Continue 6–8 or more PrescriptFit amino acid doses per day.*

- *Use PrescriptFit shakes or soups before or with meals.*

- *Use foods from Phases 2–8.*

- *Use Phase 13 foods for splurges ONLY.*

- *Take a multi-vitamin supplement.*

- *Drink 5 cups of water or calorie-free beverage daily.*

## PRESCRIPTFIT
MEDICAL NUTRITION THERAPY ▪ ▪ ▪ ▪ ▪ ▪ ▪

©2017 Stanford A. Owen, MD

toxicity, has been misinterpreted, in my opinion. The "toxic" effect of fat-carbs felt by patients is the surge of toxic cytokines and intestinal hormones flooding the bloodstream and the brain and not the effect of "gluten." Perhaps we should call them "farbs," since the combination is worse than either fat or carbs alone?

What about "whole grain" or "brown rice"? In my opinion, they are marketing gimmicks developed to distract the consumer from the harmful effect of carbohydrate. Truly "whole," uncrushed wheat will crack a tooth. Whole grain or "wild" rice is not the same as refined "brown" rice. Whole corn kernels are, indeed, whole. You will often find them in the stool intact after a "corn-on-the-cob" meal. If the grain is powdered, it is not whole grain.

Rather than get side-tracked by all the starchy food nomenclature, PrescriptFit MNT simply makes the decision, and the pleasure, simple. Eat the carb and enjoy, with or without fat. Splurge and get the urge over with.

Once your goals have been reached, Splurging twice per week will not significantly impact your health or your life. When you feel the resultant misery, simply refocus on Phase 1-8 foods and feel better.

Remember, we Western humans average 80 years of life, plus or minus 10 years. Splurging won't much shorten those life-span numbers  nor will being a perfect-diet health nut extend them much. Splurge and enjoy!

## Categories and Calories of Starches

Let's take a look at calories for different types of starches: starchy vegetables and baked goods.

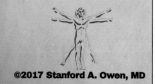

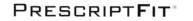

PrescriptFit®
MEDICAL NUTRITION THERAPY ▪ ▪ ▪ ▪ ▪ ▪ ▪

# ⇒ CHAPTER 7: SPLURGING ⇒

While high in calories, starchy vegetables are not all bad. Consider, for example:

> One cup of starchy vegetables equals only two ounces of beef or pork — a good caloric value.

> Two cups of beans — enough to cover an entire plate at 400 calories — is less than the calories of one donut (150 calories/oz) at 500 calories.

> Starchy vegetables are loaded with fiber and vitamins.

| STARCHY VEGETABLE | CALORIES PER CUP |
|---|---|
| Potatoes | 125 |
| Corn | 150 |
| Dried beans | 200 |
| Rice | 200 |

| BAKED GOOD | CALORIES PER OUNCE | DISTANCE TO WALK TO PAY BACK CALORIES |
|---|---|---|
| Bread (white, whole wheat, rolls, bagels, English muffins) | 80 | 1.5 miles for 1 slice of bread (150 cal.) |
| Muffins, corn bread, biscuits, pretzels, baked chips | 100 | 6–8 miles for the average muffin |
| Cereals (cold or hot) | 110 | 4 miles for a bowl of cereal plus milk |
| Pastries (donuts, Danish, croissants, crackers, cookies, cake) | 125 | 5 miles per donut; 10 miles per large cookie; 5–7 miles per slice of cake |
| Pies (all types), corn and potato chips, chocolate | 150 | 6–10 miles per slice of pie; 3 miles per 2-ounce bag of chips. |

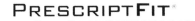

# Section B: Diving In...

Before you indulge, remember the basic principles upon which all diets are designed: People lose weight when they consume fewer calories than they need for metabolism in the organs and through physical activity. Starches may taste good, but they produce minimal satiation or fullness compared to high-protein foods. So ask yourself: Are these calories worth it or not?

Starches are the items most likely to "jump out" and grab you unexpectedly at social events, work site break rooms, or with addictive binge eating. By marking your calendar when you indulge unexpectedly in starchy foods, and by removing a planned splurge meal, you'll be able to evaluate your experience. Was that Little Debbie™ really worth removing the steak or ice cream from the calendar?

PRESCRIPTFIT®
MEDICAL NUTRITION THERAPY ■ ■ ■ ■ ■ ■ ■

# ALTERNATIVES TO FOOD PHASE STRATEGY

The most effective way to discover which foods produce symptoms or which ones "call your name" in the middle of the night is to follow the exact Food Phase strategy, either 3, 7, or 14 days in each food group before adding the next. To do so means that there will be some foods you regularly eat that you will be avoiding for several days or weeks.

*The key to your success with PrescriptFit MNT is learning what foods make you well and which ones keep you chronically ill.*

But, what if you cannot tolerate food avoidance for even one day? There are alternative solutions for you that will help you start healing, just at a slower rate than following the sequential phased approach described in this section. These alternatives let you start the PrescriptFit diet strategy in the Food Phase you feel you CAN do within the confines of your situation. These may be the most reasonable strategies for you right now!

## ALTERNATIVE SOLUTION 1: START WITH PHASE 5

If you feel like you cannot drink only shakes, soups, or puddings for even 3 days, then start in Phase 5 (PrescriptFit shakes, seafood, poultry, non-starchy vegetables, and eggs). This will give you options for breakfast that "feel" normal, such as an omelet.

If you are a fast-food junkie, starting in Phase 5 gives you options for many branded, fast-food joints that offer breakfast. It gives you options of poultry or seafood for lunch or supper, and by including vegetables, this allows you to eat salads (available everywhere) from the get-go.

Try starting in Food Phase 5 for 3, 7, or 14 days, then add one food group at a time.

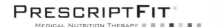

**PRESCRIPTFIT**
MEDICAL NUTRITION THERAPY

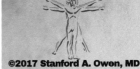

©2017 Stanford A. Owen, MD

## ALTERNATIVE SOLUTION 2: START WITH PHASE 8

Still too restrained by starting in Phase 5? Start in Food Phase 8 (PrescriptFit shakes, seafood, poultry, non-starchy vegetables, eggs, nuts, and fruit). Weight loss will be slower, but you will gain control of your medical condition relatively quickly. This alternative gives you options for snacking on nuts, fruit, and high protein snacks, and your dining options are now open to all situations, even traveling for business or vacation.

## ALTERNATIVE SOLUTION 3: ADDING PRESCRIPTFIT TO YOUR MEALS

Can't avoid carbs at all? You are probably food-addicted and require medication BUT might respond to a diet simply starting in Phase 13, with all food groups "on the table." The primary change in diet with this strategy is to ADD food into your diet in the form of PrescriptFit shakes, soups, or puddings. I recommend 6-8 doses (scoops) per day divided into morning, noon, and night. In particular, I recommend consuming PrescriptFit WITH meals as a usual component of the meal: shake, soup, or pudding (for dessert).

> **OBESITY IS NOT A CHARACTER FLAW!**
>
> You are not a better person if you can deprive yourself more than the next person.
>
> You do not have a failure in character if you require medication to avoid overeating.
>
> You do not have a failure in character if you require bariatric obesity surgery.
>
> BUT, you are a reasonable person, and effective solutions do require STRATEGY. Reasonable people can adopt strategies that are effective.

Starting in Phase 13 is not ideal, but it is an alternative that beats staying stuck with no meaningful options. The act of preparing a shake, soup, or pudding, in itself, may alter your food choices for that meal. It will probably reduce the amount you eat during the meal and it will alter how you absorb and process the meal. It will work.

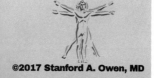

**PRESCRIPTFIT**
MEDICAL NUTRITION THERAPY ▪ ▪ ▪ ▪ ▪ ▪ ▪

## How would simply adding PrescriptFit to a meal make a meaningful difference?

PrescriptFit contains a proprietary formula of single amino acids, which are absorbed by your body's cells faster than any food (including simple sugar) that you eat. These amino acids are immediately absorbed passively through the intestinal wall. They do not require digestion or a receptor "pump" to enter the blood stream like sugars and complex carbohydrates.

Once in the blood stream in high concentrations (i.e., two scoops), the amino acids can enter cells instantly, where they can then be used for either energy (like sugar) or cellular growth and repair. This is a huge advantage over sugar or complex carbohydrate. PrescriptFit bypasses the normal digestion and metabolism pathways without the need of insulin! What results is a "damping" or diminished cascade of dangerous cytokine hormones into the bloodstream that would normally occur with a high-fat/high-carbohydrate meal. The surge of hormones, including insulin, does not occur when using the PrescriptFit amino acids. Your symptoms improve and eventually, you will see improvement in your medical measures, such as blood sugar or blood pressure.

If you are a person that simply cannot or will not avoid certain foods, consider long-term medication to improve your eating drives. Remember that being food addicted is not a character flaw; you simply have body chemistry that drives you to eat and avoid deprivation. You are certainly not alone either; you struggle with the same body chemistry issues as most humans. This is why in countries considered "developed," a majority of the population becomes overweight or obese. These high-fat, high-carbohydrate choices are on every corner, every commercial, in every magazine, and every supermarket. A regular diet of these foods leads to food addiction and obesity.

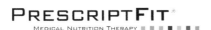

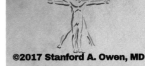

# NOTES

**QUESTIONS?**
EMAIL DR. OWEN AT
DROWENMD@DRDIET.COM

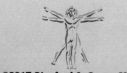

**PRESCRIPTFIT**®
MEDICAL NUTRITION THERAPY

# SECTION C

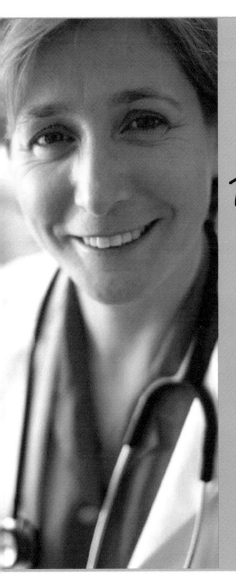

Getting
Well —
Using
PrescriptFit
to Treat
Illness

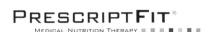

PRESCRIPTFIT®
MEDICAL NUTRITION THERAPY

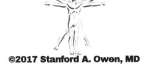

©2017 Stanford A. Owen, MD

# TABLE OF CONTENTS

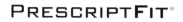

PRESCRIPT**FIT**®
MEDICAL NUTRITION THERAPY ■ ■ ■ ■ ■ ■ ■

# SECTION C: GETTING WELL — USING PRESCRIPTFIT TO TREAT ILLNESS

PrescriptFit® was developed as a way to help treat illness and chronic symptoms that keep you from feeling your best. The concept of Medical Nutrition Therapy (MNT) is about:

> **Improving your quality of life on a very basic level of wellness** — a first step toward enhancing other areas of anyone's life. It's hard to do the things you need to improve your education, your work situation, or your relationships if you just don't feel well.

> **Participating with your healthcare provider** to get the best quality medical care you can; that means you and your provider working together to diagnose and treat disease AND to measure response to treatment.

> **"Fitting" treatment for illness to the individual.** Each person's health changes as diet, age, illness, medication, or life events change. What makes your body perform at its best may be very different from those around you and at different times and during different circumstances you encounter in life.

> **Learning that disease and diet are intimately connected** AND exactly how you can balance that connection to feel better. You discover what, how, and when what you eat makes your symptoms improve or worsen.

**PrescriptFit's Medical Nutrition Therapy stresses:**

- *Actively working with your healthcare provider*

- *Using nutrition change to help treat a variety of medical conditions*

- *Discovering for yourself exactly what level or type of lifestyle change makes YOU feel better*

- *Measuring response REGULARLY to nutrition change*

**PRESCRIPTFIT**
MEDICAL NUTRITION THERAPY ▪ ▪ ▪ ▪ ▪ ▪ ▪

©2017 Stanford A. Owen, MD

# CHAPTER 8: LINKING DIET & ILLNESS

On a global scale, quality of life is defined as, "...a broad ranging concept, incorporating in a complex way individuals' physical health, psychological state, level of independence, social relationships, personal beliefs, and their relationships to salient features of the environment...quality of life is subjective, includes both positive and negative facets of life and is multi-dimensional. [The World Health Organization Quality of Life Group, 1995, p. 1405]

## QUALITY OF LIFE AND PRESCRIPTFIT

On a personal level (apart from income, social, family, and cultural issues), how we might rate our individual quality of life tends to have a lot to do with:

*Clinical experience with PrescriptFit for over 10 years has shown that MNT positively augments treatment for disorders that seriously compromise elements of daily quality of life.*

> Eating things that taste good and avoiding digestive problems, such as GERD (acid reflux) and irritable bowel syndrome

> Avoiding chronic illness, such as diabetes mellitus, hypertension, hyperlipidemia, insulin resistant syndrome (IRS or metabolic syndrome), steatosis (fatty liver)

> Feeling energetic without suffering the overall fatigue of fibromyalgia or the debilitating sadness of depression

> Moving without pain and/or swelling often associated with migraine headaches and arthritis as well as back, knee, and joint pain

> Enjoying sex instead of worrying about problems with libido, sexual dysfunction, or infertility

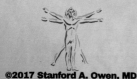

**PRESCRIPTFIT**
MEDICAL NUTRITION THERAPY ▪ ▪ ▪ ▪ ▪ ▪

> Increasing the odds of living longer by minimizing the risk of heart disease and stroke

> Breathing easy without suffering shortness of breath or asthma and allergies

> Sleeping soundly and regularly by controlling sleep apnea and insomnia

From our 10 years' clinical experience with PrescriptFit, we've found that MNT positively augments treatment for these disorders that seriously compromise the quality of life.

This chapter includes specific information about a variety of disease/symptom categories positively impacted by MNT.

Disease/Symptom Questionnaires are located following each topic to measure response after each Food Phase or every four weeks. These questionnaires also appear at the back of your PrescriptFit Calendar.

## YOU, YOUR HEALTHCARE PROVIDER, AND

*Medical textbooks cite MNT as the first line of treatment for many diseases, including:*

- *Acid reflux (GERD)*
- *Diabetes*
- *Migraines*
- *High cholesterol*
- *High blood pressure*
- *Metabolic syndrome (IRS)*
- *Irritable bowel syndrome*
- *Sleep apnea*
- *Steatosis (fatty liver)*

USE THE CHART ON THE NEXT PAGE TO QUICKLY ACCESS HOW TO APPROACH USING MNT FOR THOSE DISEASES OR SYMPTOMS THAT "FIT" FOR YOU

PRESCRIPTFIT®
MEDICAL NUTRITION THERAPY ▪ ▪ ▪ ▪ ▪ ▪ ▪

# SECTION C: GETTING WELL... ❦

| Diseases/Symptoms Impacting QoL Measures | MNT = First-line | MNT = Adjunct | MNT Supervision* |
|---|---|---|---|
| **QUALITY OF LIFE (QoL) MEASURES AND MNT TREATMENT** | | | |
| **HEALTHY DIGESTION** | | | |
| • Acid Reflux (GERD) | X | | |
| • Irritable Bowel Syndrome (IBS) | X | | |
| **RENEWED ENERGY** | | | |
| • Fatigue | | X | |
| • Fibromyalgia | | X | |
| • Depression | | X | |
| **PAIN FREEDOM/MOBILITY** | | | |
| • Migraine | X | | |
| • Arthritis | | X | |
| • Back, Knee, and Joint Pain | | X | |
| • Edema (Swelling) | | X | |
| **IMPROVED SEXUALITY** | | | |
| • Low Libido | | X | |
| • Sexual Dysfunction | | X | |
| • Infertility | | X | |
| **GOOD NIGHT'S REST** | | | |
| • Sleep Apnea/Snoring | X | | |
| • Insomnia | | X | |
| **WELL-MANAGED CHRONIC ILLNESS** | | | |
| • Diabetes Mellitus | X | | X |
| • Hypertension | X | X | X |
| • Hyperlipidemia | X | X | X |
| • Metabolic Syndrome (IRS) | X | X | |
| • Steatosis (fatty liver) | X | X | X |
| • Dyspnea (breathlessness) | | X | X |
| • Congestive Heart Failure | | X | X |
| • Angina Pectoris | | X | X |
| • Asthma | | X | X |

\* WARNING: MNT requires close medical supervision: your healthcare provider may want you to discontinue certain medications quickly if your disease symptoms subside to avoid critical problems with blood pressure or cardiac function.

**PRESCRIPTFIT**
MEDICAL NUTRITION THERAPY ▪ ▪ ▪ ▪ ▪ ▪ ▪

# CHAPTER 8: LINKING DIET & ILLNESS

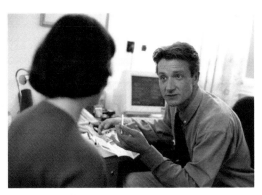

## PRESCRIPTFIT

PrescriptFit Medical Nutrition Therapy is designed to help you and your healthcare provider treat diet-responsive disease and measure results. Diet-responsive illnesses are those that positively improve when treatment includes a change in the way you eat. Every diet-responsive medical condition has specific **signs, symptoms, or measures.**

> **A sign** is something you can easily see — An increase/decrease in weight, change in waist size, swelling, changes in skin coloration (pink/gray).

> **A symptom** is something you feel — Fatigue, shortness of breath, snoring, pain, sadness, worry.

> **A measure** is something you learn from a lab text or exam procedure — Blood pressure, blood sugar count, or cholesterol level.

You may have several medical conditions present at the same time that require taking a variety of medications, even some that counteract the side effects of others. Ask your healthcare provider to help you learn to

## PRESCRIPTFIT

MEDICAL NUTRITION THERAPY

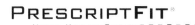

## WHAT DO I NEED TO DO?

1. Before beginning the PrescriptFit MNT Plan, visit your healthcare provider to gather the information you need to note symptoms, signs, and measures on your PrescriptFit Calendar's Disease Score Sheet. Take your Calendar with you to the appointment so you can record these findings right away. (See pages 47 through 49 for a more information on talking with your healthcare provider about the PrescriptFit MNT Plan.)

2. Re-measure each Disease Score Sheet after each Food Phase or every four weeks. If your symptoms, signs, or measures don't improve or return to a previous level, begin Food Phase 1 again and repeat the 13 Food Phases until you reach the "feel-good" point again. If you diligently adhere to PrescriptFit, diet-responsive illness should improve.

3. Fill out the PrescriptFit Quality of Life Questionnaire every 12 weeks (available for download free of charge at www.drdiet.com) until you reach what you feel to be your maximum improvement.

4. Ask your healthcare provider if further improvement is possible; then measure progress every 12 weeks indefinitely.

*The PrescriptFit Disease/Symptom Questionnaires and scoring systems are based on Dr. Owen's clinical experience from the past 10 years. These results are important primarily for what they might mean for you, and secondly for helping your healthcare provider treat your illness.*

measure each medical condition independently to better understand whether or not what you eat contributes to the problem.

Remember, a diet is something very personal. Who we are, how we feel, and how we look in size and shape are the results of what we eat, our eating habits as well as our lifestyle. If you want to change the way you FEEL, you need to find a way to change your "diet" to what your body needs to make you feel better.

With MNT, you use the number of doses of amino acids, the information you collect about how you feel, and the flexible Food Phases to design the "diet" that works best to feel better from now on.

# CHAPTER 9: MNT AS FIRST-LINE TREATMENT

**PRESCRIPTFIT**
MEDICAL NUTRITION THERAPY ▪ ▪ ▪ ▪ ▪ ▪ ▪

# CHAPTER 9: FIRST-LINE TREATMENT

MNT can be used as a first-line treatment for managing symptoms associated with:

> Acid reflux (GERD)

> Diabetes

> Migraines

> High cholesterol

> High blood pressure

> Metabolic syndrome (IRS)

> Irritable bowel syndrome

> Sleep apnea

> Steatosis (fatty liver)

Key to this treatment is keeping track of the symptoms you have, how severe they might be, and how they might change as you follow the PrescriptFit Plan. You may notice that symptoms lessen significantly in the first few phases of the Plan, but return quickly when you get to the later phases or cut back on your amino acid doses.

Following the MNT Plan also means keeping track of what medications you take (both those prescribed by your healthcare provider and those sold "over the counter") AND how often you take them. You may find that you will no longer need to take many of these medications OR take them nearly as often by following the MNT Plan.

*Measuring the symptom changes you experience will give you the DATA you need to know how to fit MNT to you. The flexibility and creativity built into the Plan gives you the POWER to make that "fit" a creative, long-term solution to feeling better.*

**WARNING:**

NEVER CHANGE HOW MUCH OR HOW OFTEN YOU TAKE ANY PRESCRIBED MEDICATION WITHOUT MEDICAL CONSULT.

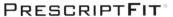

**PRESCRIPTFIT**
MEDICAL NUTRITION THERAPY ▪ ▪ ▪ ▪ ▪ ▪ ▪ ▪

©2017 Stanford A. Owen, MD

## ⁓ Section C: Getting Well... ⁓

### Acid Reflux Disease (GERD): Dyspepsia, Heartburn, Peptic Ulcers

#### What is Acid Reflux?

*Did you know?*

1. GERD is the most common ailment worldwide.

2. Antacid medication is the #1 selling class of medication.

3. The incidence of GERD has steadily increased with worldwide obesity.

*If these mechanisms can cause GERD, why do symptoms often disappear after only six weeks of a Medical Nutrition Therapy Plan? The answer is: we don't know!*

Acid reflux or GERD occurs when acid from the stomach flows backward in the "swallowing tube" or esophagus. Typically, this happens because the muscle (sphincter) that keeps the lower end of the esophagus closed once food/liquid passes through to the stomach "relaxes" more than normal. This "reflux" often causes stomach pain, heartburn, indigestion, and/or bloating; sometimes, people experience chest pain or difficulty swallowing as a result. Left untreated, GERD can cause serious damage to the esophagus.

#### What Causes GERD?

Physicians really don't know why reflux occurs more in some people than others. One cause can be mechanical — a hiatal hernia (dislocation of the stomach through the "hiatus" of the diaphragm and into the chest) allows acid to penetrate the esophagus. "Stress" causes excess acid secretion, which can make the reflux more likely and more severe. Some medications (such as those often prescribed for arthritis) can dissolve the stomach's mucous lining, allowing damaging acid to "eat away" at the stomach. Finally, we know that a bacteria named "H. Pylori" damages the protective mucous barrier and directly inflames the stomach lining.

All four mechanisms — mechanical, stress, medications, and bacteria — may be present. In addition, the interrelationship of obesity, diet, and GERD is complex and hard to define.

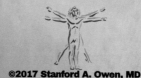

**PRESCRIPTFIT**
MEDICAL NUTRITION THERAPY ▪ ▪ ▪ ▪ ▪ ▪ ▪

# ∼ Chapter 9: First-Line Treatment ∼

## What Role Might Cytokine Imbalance Play?

One theory is that fat cell-produced cytokines influence acid secretion, inflammation, and the ability to move food/liquid through the digestive system. When cytokine-producing diets change to cytokine-balancing diets, these functions improve.

## What Results Could I Expect with MNT?

In my clinic, 67 percent of all patients at initial evaluation use some type of antacid medication for symptom relief. Within three months of beginning the PrescriptFit MNT Plan, 87 percent no longer suffer from GERD symptoms and can discontinue taking antacid medication.

## How Can I Measure Symptom Change on the Plan?

First, you need to be clear about what symptoms of GERD you might have. Next, you want to have a measurement of how severe each symptom is for you. This will give you a "baseline" to compare with future measurements. Most importantly, talk with your healthcare provider at each regular visit about your symptoms and how they might change using the PrescriptFit Plan.

> *You (and your healthcare provider) won't know how PrescriptFit is helping you without a way to measure progress.*

As with any medical condition, treatment for GERD often involves taking medications to reduce symptoms. With PrescriptFit, you may find that as your symptoms lessen, you will need to take less medication OR perhaps discontinue your medications entirely. If you are taking prescription medicines, talk to your healthcare provider about when and how to cut down on what you take BEFORE you make any changes.

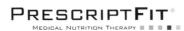

**PRESCRIPTFIT**
MEDICAL NUTRITION THERAPY ▪ ▪ ▪ ▪ ▪ ▪ ▪

©2017 Stanford A. Owen, MD

# ∼ SECTION C: GETTING WELL... ∼

## ACID REFLUX (GERD) DISEASE/SYMPTOM QUESTIONNAIRE

| Symptom Experience | Level of Discomfort | | |
|---|---|---|---|
| Heartburn | None             Severe<br>0 1 2 3 4 5 6 7 8 9 10 | | |
| Pain in pit of stomach | None             Severe<br>0 1 2 3 4 5 6 7 8 9 10 | | |
| Food/liquid in mouth during sleep | None             Severe<br>0 1 2 3 4 5 6 7 8 9 10 | | |
| Bloating after meals | None             Severe<br>0 1 2 3 4 5 6 7 8 9 10 | | |

### GERD Medications Used:
**Circle those used and frequency as indicated below.**

| Over-the-counter antacids (Maalox™, Tums™, etc.) | Daily | >2X/week | >2X/month |
|---|---|---|---|

**Prescription Medications** (Circle all taken 1+ times a week)

| | | |
|---|---|---|
| Nexium | Pepcid | Propulsid |
| Prilosec | Prevacid | Tagamet |
| Zantac | Protonix | Axid |
| Reglan | | |

Other (list) _____

\* WARNING: Never discontinue a prescribed medication without consulting your healthcare provider.

# ~ CHAPTER 9: FIRST-LINE TREATMENT ~

## TYPE 2 DIABETES
## (DIABETES MELLITUS, ADULT ONSET)

### WHAT IS TYPE 2 DIABETES?

Diabetes is a disease that results from either a failure of the pancreas' ability to produce enough insulin (a hormone that regulates how your body uses and stores nutrients) or a failure of the body's response to the insulin produced.

Diabetes is diagnosed when fasting (12-hour fast) blood glucose (known as an FPG) is 126 mg/dl or greater or the glucose level after a meal is of 200 mg/dl or greater. A "pre-diabetes" condition exists when the fasting blood sugar is 110 mg/dl or above.

### WHAT CAUSES DIABETES?

Diabetes is not just an abnormality of blood sugar. All carbohydrates (sugar), protein, and fats used in the body are under the direct control of insulin. When cells become "resistant" to the action of insulin, our bodies shut the "gates" on the surface of our cells that let sugar, protein, and fats enter the cells for processing. As a result, these nutrients accumulate in the blood stream, leading to elevated blood sugar, blood fats (cholesterol/triglycerides), and abnormal protein metabolism. Our cells try to compensate but eventually "starve" and die. The result is damage to brain and nerve cells, kidney, liver, muscle, bone, and blood vessels, which leads to dementia, neuropathy (painful nerve damage), heart attack, stroke, kidney failure (dialysis), fatty liver (cirrhosis), muscle wasting and weakness, osteoporosis, and arthritis. Those with diabetes also suffer from immune impairment, which causes a marked increase in cancer, especially breast and colon cancer.

*According to the Centers for Disease Control 2014 National Diabetes Statistics Report, 9.3 percent of Americans have diabetes, and another 27.8 percent have the disease but are likely undiagnosed.*

*PrescriptFit offers a structure for you to get control of your blood glucose levels and maintain that control over a lifetime of diabetes treatment.*

PRESCRIPTFIT
MEDICAL NUTRITION THERAPY ■ ■ ■ ■ ■ ■ ■

In addition, when cells "think" they are starving, they send messages to the pancreas to produce more insulin. As a result, the pancreas becomes exhausted from chronic insulin overproduction. "Resting" the pancreas with diet and improving muscle cell sensitivity to insulin via exercise can restore the pancreas to proper function without medication.

### What Role Might Cytokine Imbalance Play?

The impact of cytokine imbalance on insulin resistance occurs in three ways. Some cytokines promote cell "resistance" to insulin (e.g., resistin). Others directly enhance how sensitive the cell is to insulin. Still other cytokines cause further malfunction because they interfere with the production of or action of these first two types.

Because MNT both removes toxic foods and offers cells repairing amino acids, there is a marked reduction in the toxic cytokines that damage insulin receptors. Improvement in insulin receptors on the cell surface allows insulin to land (like a spaceship to a space station) to open the "gates" for the nutrients your cells need.

### What Results Could I Expect with MNT?

PrescriptFit MNT can be used to correct insulin receptor metabolism and improve type 2 diabetes symptoms by:

1. Removing the nutrients that cause insulin receptor damage: Phases 9-13 foods and sugary drinks (soda, juice, milk, and sweet tea)

2. Adding the nutrients that can be metabolized without the action of insulin or insulin receptors. Micronized amino acids, as

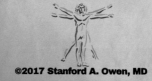

**PRESCRIPTFIT**®
MEDICAL NUTRITION THERAPY ▪ ▪ ▪ ▪ ▪ ▪ ▪

formulated in PrescriptFit products, do not require insulin because they are rapidly absorbed from the gut without digestion and pass directly into your bloodstream. Once in the blood stream in sufficient amounts, amino acids flood rapidly into cells where they can be used for energy (like sugar) or protein growth or repair, bypassing the need for insulin. Cells improve immediately.

*These improvements in cell metabolism can be realized before the prescription of any drug or medication. Medication, when necessary, can further improve insulin receptor function and cell metabolism.*

As cells recover and use insulin properly, the pancreas can recover (like a rested muscle after exercise) and start functioning more normally.

So why do doctors not initially use PrescriptFit or other Medical Nutrition Therapy strategies, as directed by textbooks, government agencies, and professional organizations? The reasons are complex:

> **Inadequate Nutrition Training** — Doctors have ZERO training in nutrition therapy either in medical school or in specialty residency training.

> **Lack of Dietician Access** — Dieticians rarely work in healthcare provider's offices and are paid little or nothing for counseling time. Most are located in higher paying hospital settings, where they virtually never follow patients over a period of years.

> **Focus on Weight Loss** — Because most diet programs focus on weight loss, both the public and physicians miss the fact that metabolism is quickly correctable. Thinking that large weight loss is necessary to control diabetes is a mistake. Weight loss is difficult. Most doctors are fatalistic about patient motivation to change diet. Most patients give up on weight loss, having "failed" in the past with dieting.

This last factor is closely related to the resistance of brain and muscle cells to insulin, which causes

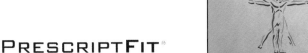

**PRESCRIPTFIT**®
MEDICAL NUTRITION THERAPY ▪ ▪ ▪ ▪ ▪ ▪ ▪

©2017 Stanford A. Owen, MD

*Study each applicable disease section, and complete the Disease/Symptom Questionnaires to track exactly how MNT helps with diabetes-related symptoms.*

a "starvation" reaction. Those with diabetes are, literally, constantly hungry for sugar. Most would describe themselves as "food addicts." Lack of knowledge on how to manage and control this "starvation metabolism" in the brain leads to both doctors and patients themselves to see a lack of "willpower" as a character flaw — an unfortunate pre-judgment (prejudice). Strategies exist to resolve this dilemma with both nutrition and medication.

Many people with diabetes, experience something called "diabetic neuropathy," which is nerve damage, frequently described as burning in the feet or legs. These symptoms typically improve, especially if present for only a few years. Other conditions related to diabetes usually improve with MNT as well, including: hypertension, edema (swelling), elevated cholesterol/triglycerides, sleep disorders, fatigue, and depression.

### HOW CAN I MEASURE SYMPTOM CHANGE ON THE PLAN?

You need to be clear about whether or not you have type 2/adult onset diabetes mellitus. If monitoring blood sugar with a home test kit (available at pharmacies), record daily glucose readings until they are normal and stay normal (FPG level at less than 126 mg/dl).  If you currently take medications for diabetes, your healthcare provider should closely supervise your treatment throughout the MNT Plan. If you don't currently take diabetes medications, talk to your healthcare provider about planning 12 weeks of PrescriptFit MNT before prescribing these medications.

*In our clinic, 90 percent of patients with diabetes gain control of their condition if they precisely follow the 14-day Plan. By restarting Food Phase 1 each time you "go off" the plan, you can regain and maintain glucose control.*

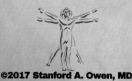

PRESCRIPTFIT
MEDICAL NUTRITION THERAPY ▪ ▪ ▪ ▪ ▪ ▪ ▪

# CHAPTER 9: FIRST-LINE TREATMENT

## WHAT DO I NEED TO DO?

1. Clear the house all diabetes-causing foods (sugary drinks and Phases 9-13 foods).

2. Improve your cell function immediately with PrescriptFit micronized amino acid products.

3. Add foods that are not likely to provoke insulin resistance and diabetes (Phases 2-8).

4. Monitor daily blood glucose with a home testing kit.

5. Have your healthcare provider complete the lab test portions of the Disease/Symptom Questionnaire below before you begin MNT and every 12 weeks thereafter.

6. Record any symptoms you have related to circulatory problems associated with diabetes.

7. Indicate how many medications you currently take for diabetes.

8. Keep track of your subjective (symptoms) and objective (FPG and A1C) findings after each Food Phase.

9. Review the results with your healthcare provider during each visit. Talk about how you're feeling and whether or not you might need to alter the type or dose of medications you currently take for your diabetes.

10. ONCE DIABETES IS CONTROLLED, add toxic foods of Phases 9-13 in a managed strategy of Splurging twice per week (more or less).

## DIABETES (TYPE 2) DISEASE/SYMPTOM QUESTIONNAIRE

| Fasting Blood Sugar* | Hemoglobin A1C* |
|---|---|
| Initial____   12-Week____ | Initial____   12-Week____ |
| **Neuropathy Present** | **Neuropathy at 12 Weeks** |
| Burning legs/feet<br>　　　　　yes___ no___<br>Restless legs yes___ no___<br>Numbness yes___ no___ | Burning legs/feet<br>　　　　　yes___ no___<br>Restless legs yes___ no___<br>Numbness yes___ no___ |

\* Hemoglobin A1C kits and home glucose kits are available at all pharmacies.

**Number of Diabetes Medications Used ____**
**(e.g., glyburide + metformin = 2)**

\* WARNING: Never discontinue a prescribed medication without consulting with your healthcare provider

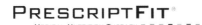

**PRESCRIPTFIT**
MEDICAL NUTRITION THERAPY ▪ ▪ ▪ ▪ ▪ ▪ ▪

©2017 Stanford A. Owen, MD

# ⸙ Section C: Getting Well... ⸙

## Headache (from Migraine, Muscle Tension, and "Pseudotumor")

### What is Headache?

*The most common types of chronic headache — migraine, muscle tension, and pseudotumor — all respond to the MNT Plan for different reasons and at different rates.*

Headache is a common symptom that may result from a number of different problems or illnesses. Headaches are classified as either "primary" or "secondary." Primary headaches are those that occur without appearing to be caused by another illness such as tension headaches or migraines. Secondary headaches can result from a number of conditions, ranging from life-threatening brain tumors, strokes, and meningitis to less-serious (but common) problems people experience when they stop ingesting caffeine or discontinue some pain-killing medication.

### What Causes Migraine, Muscle Tension, and Pseudotumor-related Headaches?

*Migraine is often commonly mistaken for "sinus" headache, since migraine often causes congestion. If the throbbing of the headache is sensitive to light or sound OR gets worse when bending or stooping, it is probably migraine.*

**Migraine** is a throbbing headache usually originating in the front or side of the head. Its cause is unknown; however, a number of "triggers" have been identified such as stress, sleep disturbances, hormones, bright or flickering lights, certain odors, cigarette smoke, alcohol, aged cheeses, chocolate, monosodium glutamate, nitrites, and caffeine.

**Pseudotumor cerebri** is a condition due to excess spinal fluid pressure; it is most common in people who gain weight and become obese, especially women. The cause is unknown.

**Muscle tension headaches** can be related to posture problems that occur in those with large abdomens or breasts and improve with treatment for the neck muscles involved. Muscle tension or traction headaches from excess weight may take longer to resolve and relate to total weight loss.

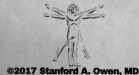

**PRESCRIPTFIT**®
MEDICAL NUTRITION THERAPY ■ ■ ■ ■ ■ ■ ■

# CHAPTER 9: FIRST-LINE TREATMENT

## WHAT ROLE MIGHT CYTOKINE IMBALANCE PLAY?

**Migraine** is due to swelling and inflammation of brain blood vessels. This swelling and inflammation cause irritation of brain nerve fibers which then convey pain across the head and face. The swelling and inflammation are mediated by proteins in the cytokine class. As in other illness, genetic factors play a role. It is possible the inflammatory and swelling related cytokines generated from fat cells, liver, and intestine contribute to these genetic migraine triggers in obesity.

*Because migraine is 500 percent more common in obesity (although the reason is unknown), MNT is considered a first-line treatment.*

Why **pseudotumor** responds to MNT is also unknown. Hormones and cytokine proteins control spinal fluid regulation in the brain. Cytokines from fat tissue may influence formation or removal of spinal fluid. Only a spinal puncture can diagnose pseudotumor. If headache responds to the PrescriptFit MNT Plan, pseudotumor should be considered likely, even without a spinal puncture.

*MNT is the recommended first-line treatment of pseudotumor to decrease spinal fluid pressure.*

Since pseudotumor predominately affects women, hormones obviously play a role. Exactly how fat-produced cytokines and hormones interplay to prevent removal of spinal fluid is unknown. However, it is likely that cytokines mediate the process. Why? Because headache improves and pressure measures from spinal puncture register decreases in days or weeks after starting PrescriptFit Plan, long before substantial weight loss occurs.

**Muscle tension headache** will only improve at the rate that the mechanical strain that causes it improves. Weight loss and decreased inflammation will help alleviate mechanical strain sooner. Headaches that improve rapidly on the Plan are probably due to another cause.

PRESCRIPTFIT
MEDICAL NUTRITION THERAPY ■ ■ ■ ■ ■ ■ ■

©2017 Stanford A. Owen, MD

# ⌒ SECTION C: GETTING WELL... ⌒

*The diet control and design of PrescriptFit Plan allows a more objective way to evaluate the role of diet and obesity on headache.*

## WHAT RESULTS COULD I EXPECT WITH MNT?

Clinical experience with MNT and headache varies with the cause. **Pseudotumor** responds within days or weeks but requires a spinal puncture for confirmation. **Migraine** may respond quickly; however, it has many triggers and a naturally variable course. Therefore, long-term response can be gauged only by recording headache scores on the Disease/Symptom Questionnaire over time (e.g., monthly for at least a year). **Muscle tension headache** should respond based on total weight loss.

## HOW CAN I MEASURE SYMPTOM CHANGE ON THE PLAN?

First, you need to be clear about what may be causing your headaches. If your headache is caused by another medical condition or situation (e.g., caffeine withdrawal), work with your healthcare provider to identify the source and plan appropriate treatment. Next, you want to measure how severe each symptom is for you. This will give you a "baseline" to compare with future measurements.

*Some people suffer with all three types of headache. Note when and how much your headache improves as well as whether or not headaches return during a particular Food Phase. If this happens, go back to the previous Food Phase and note what happens. If you can't identify a specific Food Phase that relates to the headache returning, start Phase 1 again and proceed forward until you identify a pattern.*

Most importantly, you (and your healthcare provider) need a way to measure progress over time. Talk with your provider at each regular visit about your symptoms and how they might change using the Plan.

As with any medical condition, treatment traditionally means taking medications to reduce symptoms. A number of prescription and over-the-counter medications help alleviate headache pain and, in the case of migraine, provide some prevention. With this Plan, you may find that as symptoms lessen, you need less medication. If you are taking prescription medicines, talk to your healthcare provider about when and how to cut down on what you take BEFORE you make any changes.

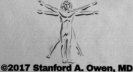

# PRESCRIPTFIT
MEDICAL NUTRITION THERAPY ▪ ▪ ▪ ▪ ▪ ▪ ▪

# ⚘ CHAPTER 9: FIRST-LINE TREATMENT ⚘

## WHAT DO I NEED TO DO?

1. Check each symptom you are currently experiencing in the Disease/ Symptom Questionnaire below.

2. Grade the level of discomfort you have on a scale from 0–10 (with "0" being no symptom at all to a "10" being severe discomfort) as well as how often you need medication for the pain.

3. Be sure to check the symptoms and grade your level of discomfort AGAIN at the end of each Food Phase or every four weeks.

4. Total the number of medications you currently take for headache, and check the names of any you recognize. Be sure to re-record this information at the end of each Food Phase or every four weeks.

5. Take the results with you to your next medical appointment. Talk about how you're feeling and whether or not you still need any prescription medications for headache.

### HEADACHE DISEASE/SYMPTOM QUESTIONNAIRE

| Headache Symptoms | Level of Discomfort | |
|---|---|---|
| Frequency | **None**        **Constant/Daily** <br> 0 1 2 3 4 5 6 7 8 9 10 | |
| Severity (Average) | **Mild**        **Severe** <br> 0 1 2 3 4 5 6 7 8 9 10 | |
| Medication Required | **Never**        **Always** <br> 0 1 2 3 4 5 6 7 8 9 10 | |

### Headache Medications Used: Check medications used on a daily basis and total (e.g., aspirin + Tylenol = 2)

**Medications** (Check all applicable. Total medications = \_\_\_)

- ☐ **Aspirin**
- ☐ **Acetaminophen (Tylenol™)**
- ☐ **NSAIDS (ibuprofen, naproxen, Celebrex™, Bextra™, other)**
- ☐ **Tryptan (Imitrex™, Relpax™, Maxalt™, Zomig™, other)**
- ☐ **Anti-seizure (Depakote™, Topamax™, Zonegran™, Neurontin™, Gabatril™, Tegretol™, other)**
- ☐ **Opiates (propoxephene, hydrocodone, meperidine) — Lorcet™, Vicodan™, Oxycontin™, etc.**
- ☐ **Injectable medication at hospital or clinic**

\* WARNING: Never discontinue a prescribed medication without consulting with your healthcare provider.

## PRESCRIPTFIT®
MEDICAL NUTRITION THERAPY ∎ ∎ ∎ ∎ ∎ ∎ ∎

## HYPERLIPIDEMIA (ELEVATED CHOLESTEROL AND/OR TRIGLYCERIDES)

### WHAT IS HYPERLIPIDEMIA?

*The seven- and 14-day Food Phases should be used when treating cholesterol or triglycerides with the MNT Plan.*

Hyperlipidemia is literally the presence of too much fat in the bloodstream. With this condition, you will have elevated cholesterol counts (LDL, HDL, and total cholesterol) and/or triglycerides. Excess levels of these fats speed up the process of hardening of the arteries, which reduces blood flow and can cause heart attack or stroke.

Lowering cholesterol and triglyceride levels decreases this risk. Although some experts believe that current guidelines are not conservative enough, physicians recommend that, to minimize your risk of heart disease, your desirable lipid levels should be:

> LDL less than 130 mg/dL (ideal less than 70)

> HDL greater than 40 mg/dL (men) or 50 mg/dL (women)

> Total cholesterol less than 200 mg/dL (ideal less than 150)

> Triglycerides less than 150 mg/dL

Medications are often required to achieve these levels; however, therapeutic lifestyle changes (TLC), including healthy diet and exercise choices, are considered the first line of treatment.

*Hyperlipidemia is the single greatest risk factor for heart disease, although many individuals with "normal" cholesterol levels can develop blockage.*

Elevated cholesterol levels do not absolutely predict blockage. Imaging technology may help measure degree of artery blockage. Carotid artery ultrasound and coronary artery calcium deposits can be measured. Coronary calcium scoring is more expensive, and it requires a CT scan.

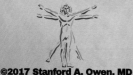

PRESCRIPTFIT
MEDICAL NUTRITION THERAPY ▪ ▪ ▪ ▪ ▪ ▪ ▪

# CHAPTER 9: FIRST-LINE TREATMENT

## WHAT CAUSES HYPERLIPIDEMIA?

There are two types of hyperlipidemia:

> **The type that runs in families.** If a close relative had early heart disease (father or brother affected before age 55, mother or sister affected before age 65), you also have an increased risk.

> **The type caused by lifestyle habits or treatable medical conditions.** Lifestyle-related causes include obesity, being sedentary, and smoking. Medical conditions that cause hyperlipidemia include diabetes, kidney disease, pregnancy, and having an underactive thyroid gland.

*Age can contribute to risk as well — men over 45 and women over 55 are more likely to develop hyperlipidemia.*

## WHAT ROLE MIGHT CYTOKINE IMBALANCE PLAY?

The study of atherosclerosis (hardening of the arteries) is now focused primarily in inflammation of the arteries rather than nutritional overload of the bloodstream with fat (although both are important). Cytokines are the primary mediator of inflammation and the focus of most research now is how to reduce cytokine-induced inflammation damage to the arteries. Inflammation leads to cholesterol deposits within the artery, collagen damage resulting in "hardening" or calcification of the artery, and clotting on the damaged surface of the inflamed artery. Diet plays a role in promoting or reducing the degree of inflammation cytokines produce. PrescriptFit optimizes protection from excess cytokine production.

## WHAT RESULTS COULD I EXPECT WITH MNT?

For most of our patients, Food Phases 1 and 2 are associated with the most profound decreases in cholesterol and triglyceride levels. You may see

**PRESCRIPTFIT**
MEDICAL NUTRITION THERAPY ▪ ▪ ▪ ▪ ▪ ▪ ▪ ▪

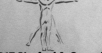

# ~ Section C: Getting Well... ~

rises in cholesterol levels with some Food Phases that involve some saturated fats, such as those that allow poultry, eggs, pork, beef, dairy, or baked goods. Nuts may actually lower cholesterol levels.

Proving you can control cholesterol with diet, then demonstrating which foods elevate cholesterol, makes infinitely more sense than initially taking a cholesterol-lowering medication. Even if medication is required, diet management is still very important. The learning curve provided by the MNT Plan can be invaluable in deciding if a particular food should be avoided or medication required.

## How Can I Measure Lipid Change on the Plan?

First, talk to your healthcare provider about your cholesterol and triglyceride levels as well as your risk level, in general, for heart disease. Have your provider share with you what your last "lipids screening" results were. This will give you a "baseline" to compare with future measurements. Next, purchase a cholesterol testing kit at a local pharmacy (available without a prescription). Test your cholesterol levels every four weeks if using the recommended 7- or 14-day Plans.

Most importantly, you (and your provider) need a way to measure progress over time. Discuss at each regular medical visit your symptoms and how they might change using the PrescriptFit Plan. Share your test results with your healthcare provider.

As with any medical condition, treatment may mean that you are taking medications to reduce your cholesterol. With MNT, you may find that as symptoms lessen, you need less medication. If taking prescription medicines, talk to your healthcare provider about when and how to cut down on what you take BEFORE you make any changes.

# PRESCRIPTFIT
MEDICAL NUTRITION THERAPY ▪ ▪ ▪ ▪ ▪ ▪ ▪

# CHAPTER 9: FIRST-LINE TREATMENT

## WHAT DO I NEED TO DO?

1. Have the healthcare provider take baseline measurements indicated on the Disease/Symptom Questionnaire below.

2. Purchase a home cholesterol testing kit, and record your results at the end of each Food Phase and 12 weeks after beginning the PrescriptFit Plan.

3. Note how each food phase impacts your test results; use this knowledge to determine which food groups might best be avoided.

4. Review the results with your healthcare provider — talk about how you're feeling and whether or not you still need any prescription medications for hyperlipidemia.

### HYPERLIPIDEMIA DISEASE/SYMPTOM QUESTIONNAIRE

| Food Phase | Total Cholesterol | LDL | HDL | Triglycerides |
|---|---|---|---|---|
| Baseline Levels | | | | |
| Food Phase 1 | | | | |
| Food Phase 2 | | | | |
| Food Phase 3 | | | | |
| Food Phase 4 | | | | |
| Food Phase 5 | | | | |
| Food Phase 6 | | | | |
| Food Phase 7 | | | | |
| Food Phase 8 | | | | |
| Food Phase 9 | | | | |
| Food Phase 10 | | | | |
| Food Phase 11 | | | | |
| Food Phase 12 | | | | |
| Food Phase 13 | | | | |
| Maintenance | | | | |

\* WARNING: Never discontinue a prescribed medication without consulting with your healthcare provider.

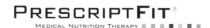

PRESCRIPTFIT®
MEDICAL NUTRITION THERAPY ▪ ▪ ▪ ▪ ▪ ▪ ▪

©2017 Stanford A. Owen, MD

# ⌐ SECTION C: GETTING WELL... ⌐

## HYPERTENSION (HIGH BLOOD PRESSURE)

### WHAT IS HYPERTENSION?

*Expert guidelines on what actually constitutes "high" blood pressure are when the systolic measurement is above 140 and the diastolic rate is above 90, expressed as 140/90. For those with diabetes or metabolic syndrome (IRS), the goal should be 130/80.*

Hypertension or high blood pressure is a condition that signals an overworking heart. Blood pressure is the result of the heart pumping blood into the arteries and the arterial blood vessels exerting resistance to the blood flow from the heart. When either of these forces — diastolic blood pressure (when the heart is resting) or systolic blood pressure (when the heart is beating) is elevated, the heart and arteries have to work under a greater strain. This can cause heart attack, stroke, kidney failure, eye disease, and atherosclerosis (hardening of the arteries). Without treatment, the heart has to work even harder to meet the blood supply needs of the body's organs and tissues, eventually resulting in cardiac disease.

### WHAT CAUSES HYPERTENSION?

There are numerous "primary" factors that can cause hypertension, including obesity, overuse of alcohol, high salt diets, aging, lack of exercise, stress, low potassium, magnesium and calcium intake, and resistance to insulin. Less common is secondary high blood pressure, which occurs as a result of a medication of some other disease (e.g., tumor).

### WHAT ROLE MIGHT CYTOKINES PLAY?

For hypertension associated with being overweight or obese, MNT is the first line of treatment because of the direct link between cytokine imbalance and weight loss. Cytokines affect salt and water retention, blood vessel spasm, clotting, and cause direct damage to the collagen structure of blood vessels. Each of these factors alone can

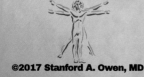

PRESCRIPTFIT
MEDICAL NUTRITION THERAPY ▪ ▪ ▪ ▪ ▪ ▪ ▪

contribute to hypertension. All of these factors work together to accelerate hypertension. MNT affects all cytokine components. Therefore, patients with hypertension lose fluid, relax blood vessels, lessen the risk of blood clots, and decrease damage to collagen. MNT is, therefore, a primary treatment of hypertension.

## WHAT RESULTS COULD I EXPECT WITH MNT?

Based on clinical experience for the past decade, the PrescriptFit MNT Plan helps patients reduce their need for antihypertensive medication. Because response is typically quite rapid, usually in Food Phase 1 and 2, you must keep in close contact with your healthcare provider to avoid medication impacts when the symptoms they treat no longer persist. Close vigilance is required to avoid hypotension (low blood pressure), especially in those using diuretics (fluid-reducing medications), or vasodilators (calcium blockers, alpha blockers).

Unless life threatening, talk to your healthcare provider about controlling your hypertension without medication using MNT. Even if medication is required initially to control high blood pressure, MNT use may very well be all you need to later discontinue or at least decrease the medication you take.

*Medical supervision is mandatory, especially in the early Food Phases of the MNT Plan.*

Start out on either the one- or two-week per Food Phase plan, especially if you taking high blood pressure medication. By adding each Food Phase at these intervals, you are more likely to identify particular food groups that contribute to hypertension.

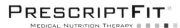

# ⌁ Section C: Getting Well... ⌁

*Pay special attention to your blood pressure during Food Phase 3 (adding poultry with saturated fat and salt used for taste) and Food Phase 6 (especially for salted nuts). You may need to cook your poultry differently and look for unsalted nuts.*

## How Can I Measure Symptom Change on the Plan?

First, you need to be clear about what may be causing your hypertension, especially if it is a secondary problem caused by another medical illness. Talk with your healthcare provider about the cause of your hypertension, possible medication therapy, and what effects MNT may have on that treatment.

Next, you want to take your blood pressure daily. Purchase a home blood pressure monitor and use it at the same time every day, preferably upon waking. This will give you a "baseline" to track improvement or change over time.

Most importantly, you need to work closely with your healthcare provider to balance medications with symptom reduction. Do NOT discontinue or change the way you take prescription medications without consulting with your healthcare provider.

## Matt — Hypertension Resolved

Matt was 44 when he came into my office in bad shape. He was severely short of breath and swollen in both legs to a point where fluid was oozing through the skin. He had the "gallop" sound of a failing heart, an elevated amount of a heart failure enzyme (BNP), with his heart putting out only half of its normal volume (an ejection fraction of 35 percent). He refused hospitalization since he would lose his job as a truck driver if he couldn't work. His blood pressure was 220/120, and his pulse was 120 with no sign of a heart attack based on his EKG.

I put Matt on PrescriptFit products for the next week. In only that first week, he lost 20 pounds of fluid buildup and then lost 44 pounds by day 16. At the end of six weeks, Matt had lost 63 pounds, 50 of which were due to fluid. His blood pressure came down to 140/70, his pulse was at 80, his feet were no longer swollen, and his heart failure was reversing. By the 12th week after that first visit to my office, his blood pressure was 120/80, BNP (that heart failure enzyme) was normal, and his heart ejection fraction had thankfully increased to 65 percent. His only treatment? Medical Nutrition Therapy with PrescriptFit products and strategies. His hypertension has remained controlled without medication.

**CASE STUDY**

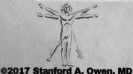

© 2017 Stanford A. Owen, MD

# PRESCRIPTFIT
MEDICAL NUTRITION THERAPY ▪ ▪ ▪ ▪ ▪ ▪ ▪

# CHAPTER 9: FIRST-LINE TREATMENT

## WHAT DO I NEED TO DO?

1. Find out if your hypertension results from weight or other diet/lifestyle-related causes.

2. Record your blood pressure at the end of each Food Phase and during the maintenance period after the last Phase (minimum of every 12 weeks).

3. Share the results you've recorded with your healthcare provider. Talk about how you're feeling and whether or not you still need any prescription medications for hypertension.

### HYPERTENSION DISEASE/SYMPTOM QUESTIONNAIRE

| Food Phase | Systolic Blood Pressure (Average) | Diastolic Blood Pressure (Average) |
|---|---|---|
| Baseline Levels | | |
| Food Phase 1 | | |
| Food Phase 2 | | |
| Food Phase 3 | | |
| Food Phase 4 | | |
| Food Phase 5 | | |
| Food Phase 6 | | |
| Food Phase 7 | | |
| Food Phase 8 | | |
| Food Phase 9 | | |
| Food Phase 10 | | |
| Food Phase 11 | | |
| Food Phase 12 | | |
| Food Phase 13 | | |
| Maintenance | | |

\* WARNING: Never discontinue a prescribed medication without consulting with your healthcare provider.

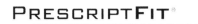

PRESCRIPTFIT®
MEDICAL NUTRITION THERAPY ▪ ▪ ▪ ▪ ▪ ▪ ▪

©2017 Stanford A. Owen, MD

# ⌐ Section C: Getting Well... ⌐

## Metabolic Syndrome (Insulin Resistant Syndrome or IRS )

### What is Insulin/Insulin Resistance?

*The PrescriptFit MNT Plan is an effective, safe, and rational way to improve insulin resistance. The Plan is first line treatment of IRS.*

Insulin is a hormone manufactured in the pancreas and released into the bloodstream when you consume carbohydrates, fats, and protein. Insulin regulates how your body metabolizes carbohydrate, fat, and protein by allowing these nutrients into your cells. The amount of insulin released is finely controlled by a feedback messaging system that relays how quickly and effectively nutrients enter individual cells (especially in the liver and muscle).

If the receptor at the cell surface no longer "allows" insulin to "land" on the cell, excess insulin accumulates in the bloodstream. Despite this overabundance of insulin in the bloodstream, the pancreas "thinks" that your body needs more insulin because the relay system isn't working properly and produces and secretes even more. This "resistance" to the action of insulin is known as the insulin resistant syndrome (or IRS).

Other terms related to IRS include "prediabetes" and "metabolic syndrome"; however, these terms mean slightly different things.

> **Prediabetes** is defined as a time period (perhaps lasting years or decades) prior to a diagnosis of diabetes when insulin metabolism is unhealthy. After years or decades of overwork, the pancreas becomes "exhausted" from the excess insulin production and fails. The result is Type 2 diabetes mellitus (thus giving rise to the term, "prediabetes").

> **Metabolic syndrome** is defined as a group of conditions (i.e., type 2 diabetes,

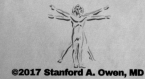

**PRESCRIPTFIT**®
MEDICAL NUTRITION THERAPY ▪ ▪ ▪ ▪ ▪ ▪ ▪

obesity, high blood pressure, and cholesterol problems) that place people at high risk for coronary artery disease. All of the conditions in this group are related to having excess insulin in the bloodstream, which causes defects, especially to adipose tissue and muscle.

Long before obvious diabetes develops, elevated insulin levels in the bloodstream can lead to abnormal metabolism, causing a number of different medical conditions — hypertension (high blood pressure), hyperlipidemia (elevated cholesterol and triglycerides), fatty liver (steatosis), sleep disorders, infertility, and depression. Although IRS can be defined as a cluster of abnormalities (e.g., obesity, hypertension, etc.) associated with insulin resistance and over-secretion of insulin by the pancreas, a cause-and-effect relationship between insulin resistance and the development of these diseases has yet to be conclusively demonstrated.

## WHAT DETERMINES IF YOU HAVE IRS?

Physicians determine if patients might have IRS by looking for any three of the following:

> **Large waist size:** Does your waist measure more than 35 inches (females) or more than 40" (males)?

> **Blood pressure:** Is your blood pressure greater than 130 systolic/85 diastolic?

> **Fasting blood sugar (FPG):** Do the results of the blood sugar test your healthcare provider runs indicate a blood sugar rate higher than 110?

> **Fasting triglycerides:** Do the results of a lipid screening indicate that blood levels of triglycerides are greater than 150?

*Additional IRS warning signs include:*

- *Thick neck*

- *Skin tags around the neck, arm pit, groin, and face*

- *Darkening and thickening of the skin of the neck, arm pit, groin, knuckles, elbows, knees, and feet*

- *Elevated blood insulin levels*

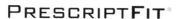

**PRESCRIPTFIT**
MEDICAL NUTRITION THERAPY ▪ ▪ ▪ ▪ ▪ ▪ ▪

> **HDL cholesterol:** Is your HDL cholesterol at an unhealthy level — less than 40 (for men) or 50 (for women)?

## WHAT ROLE MIGHT CYTOKINE IMBALANCE PLAY?

A cytokine manufactured by fat tissue, called adiponectin, is the primary factor preventing insulin resistance. Decreasing adiponectin levels are associated with increasing insulin levels and diminished insulin function. Diets high in calories, saturated or trans fats, and simple carbohydrate lower adiponectin levels, causing insulin resistance.

Another cytokine manufactured by fat tissue, resistin, causes lower adiponectin levels. Resistin also inhibits the function of insulin on cell surfaces. Elevated resistin secretion is seen in diets high in calories, saturated or trans fats, and simple carbohydrate.

Many fat- and liver-produced cytokines affect adiponectin and resistin levels. Understanding the intricacies of cytokine balance with nutrition is in the earliest phases.

Because having excess adipose (fat) tissue negatively affects how your body regulates insulin production and metabolism, losing weight on a safe, easy-to-follow plan like MNT can't help but ensure success reducing IRS symptoms. Additionally, the overproduction of cytokines due to excess adipose tissue will likely be reduced by the action of the branched-chain amino acids in PrescriptFit shakes and soups.

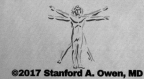

# CHAPTER 9: FIRST-LINE TREATMENT

## WHAT RESULTS COULD I EXPECT WITH MNT?

Based on our clinical experience, insulin resistance gets better in days to weeks in patients using the Prescript Fit MNT Plan. Although the mechanism for how this occurs is unclear, the result is improved sugar metabolism, lower cholesterol, and lower blood pressure.

## HOW CAN I MEASURE SYMPTOM CHANGE ON THE PLAN?

Note that some measurements associated with monitoring IRS must be done by your healthcare provider or in a health care setting, especially tests for cholesterol and blood sugar levels in your bloodstream. Of course, you can monitor your waist size, weight, and blood pressure at home.

First, have your healthcare provider share with you what measurements indicate that you have IRS from the Disease/Symptom Questionnaire on the next page. This will give you a "baseline" to compare with future measurements.

Most importantly, you (and your provider) need a way to measure progress over time. Talk with your healthcare provider at each regular visit about your symptoms and how they might change using the PrescriptFit Plan. Be sure to have your healthcare provider take the same measurements after 12 weeks on the MNT Plan as you took at the beginning.

As with any medical condition, treatment may mean that you are taking medications to reduce symptoms associated with IRS (e.g., hypertension). With PrescriptFit, you may find that as your symptoms lessen, you will need to take less medication OR perhaps discontinue your medications entirely. If you are taking prescription medicines, talk to your healthcare provider about when and how to cut down on what you take BEFORE you make any changes.

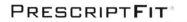

**PRESCRIPTFIT**
MEDICAL NUTRITION THERAPY ▪ ▪ ▪ ▪ ▪ ▪ ▪ ▪

©2017 Stanford A. Owen, MD

# ~ SECTION C: GETTING WELL... ~

| IRS Disease/Symptom Questionnaire | | |
|---|---|---|
| **Disease Measures** | **Baseline** | **End of Phase 12\*** |
| **Blood Pressure (systolic/diastolic)** | _____/_____ | _____/_____ |
| **Fasting Plasma Glucose** | _____mg/dL | _____mg/dL |
| **Fasting triglycerides** | _____mg/dL | _____mg/dL |
| **Waist Circumference** | _____inches | _____inches |
| **C-peptide Insulin Level** | _____mg/dL | _____mg/dL |
| **Skin Tags (Yes or No)** | _____ | _____ |
| **Acanthosis\*\* (Yes or No)** | _____ | _____ |

\* Those with IRS may not be able to do Food Phase 13 due to carbohydrate restrictions.

\*\* Dark discoloration and thickened skin of neck, axilla, elbows, knuckles, feet

\* WARNING: Never discontinue a prescribed medication without consulting with your healthcare provider.

©2017 Stanford A. Owen, MD

**PRESCRIPTFIT**
MEDICAL NUTRITION THERAPY ▪ ▪ ▪ ▪ ▪ ▪ ▪

# CHAPTER 9: FIRST-LINE TREATMENT

## IRRITABLE BOWEL SYNDROME (IBS)

### WHAT IS IRRITABLE BOWEL SYNDROME (IBS)?

IBS is one of the more common maladies affecting adults. As the name implies, IBS feels like the bowel is irritable or "angry." People with IBS experience cramps, diarrhea, feelings of constipation, and generalized abdominal pain usually experienced in the lower abdomen. "Bloating" is a common complaint, especially after meals.

### WHAT CAUSES IBS?

There may be several causes for IBS. One of the more common is the inability to digest certain sugars, which ferment because of the bacteria present in the digestive tract into the gases methane, butane, and formate. These gases are irritating to the gut, produce abnormal motility, and are quite smelly (they are components of "swamp gas" and are quite flammable). These gases have also been associated with generalized muscle pain (similar to fibromyalgia).

You should see your healthcare provider about any ongoing abdominal pain. You will probably need to have some diagnostic tests performed to rule out serious gut disease: peptic ulcers, cancer, ulcerative colitis, or Crohn's Disease (ileitis).

### WHAT ROLE MIGHT CYTOKINE IMBALANCE PLAY?

Cytokines probably play a minimal role in IBS, although the relationship to diet and gut hormone production is being studied. We know that specific gut hormones [e.g., cholecystokinin (CCK), ghrelin, motilin, gastrin] are released in different amounts and patterns depending on meal consistency. We also know that inflammatory cytokines are related to an abnormal amount or pattern of gut hormone

*All adults over 50 should have a baseline colonoscopy (and follow up every 10 years thereafter) to detect colon cancer in early stages, while still curable. Colonoscopy should be performed earlier if one has a strong family history of colon cancer, if bleeding has occurred, or if symptoms do not improve.*

*If you suspect that you have IBS, you should probably use the 7-day MNT Plan, adding Food Phases every week. This allows enough time to clearly distinguish what foods are "offenders" to IBS.*

PRESCRIPTFIT
MEDICAL NUTRITION THERAPY ▪ ▪ ▪ ▪ ▪ ▪ ▪

©2017 Stanford A. Owen, MD

# ∽ SECTION C: GETTING WELL... ∽

release. However, no consistent cause-effect relationship has yet been established.

### WHAT RESULTS COULD I EXPECT WITH MNT?

This Plan is an ideal way to test for and improve symptoms of IBS. Many patients improve or resolve using PrescriptFit strategies without the need for costly tests or medication. In our clinical experience, most patients report rapid results, often noting improvements the first week.

*While the plan may be boring for a couple of weeks, most patients with troublesome IBS find the boredom worth the effort.*

Food Phase 1 requires use of PrescriptFit lactose-free products only (no other food). You should take at least eight doses per day along with a complete multivitamin. One cannot "overdose" on PrescriptFit lactose-free products if needed to alleviate hunger.

If you are taking medication, especially for high blood pressure, diabetes, acid reflux, or cardiac disease, your healthcare provider will need to carefully monitor your condition throughout the Plan.

Food Phases likely to cause symptom recurrence are vegetables, fruit, dairy products, and starchy foods. Sugars found in milk, fruit, beans (legumes), and wheat "ferment" in the gut to form methane, butane, and formate. By adding each food group sequentially, you can identify and then avoid the offending foods. Use this four-step, "trial-and-error" approach to "weed out" the foods that make you feel bad:

*Because IBS is not a harmful condition, experimenting with offending foods will cause no harm; it will only help make changes that eliminate irritating symptoms.*

1. If symptoms increase during a particular Food Phase, simply skip that phase.

2. Add Phases and note symptoms.

3. If symptoms occur in subsequent Food Phases, skip those phases as well until all 13 Food Phases are complete.

4. Sequentially add previously offensive Food Phases and note results.

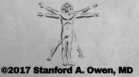

**PRESCRIPTFIT**®
MEDICAL NUTRITION THERAPY ∎ ∎ ∎ ∎ ∎ ∎ ∎

# ≈ CHAPTER 9: FIRST-LINE TREATMENT ≈

## How Can I Measure Symptom Change on the PrescriptFit Plan?

First, you need to be clear about what symptoms of IBS you might have. Next, you want to measure how severe each symptom is for you. This will give you a "baseline" to compare with future measurements. Most importantly, you (and your provider) need a way to measure progress over time. Talk with your healthcare provider at each regular visit about your symptoms and how they might change using the PrescriptFit Plan.

*The simplicity of the PrescriptFit IBS approach is that one group of foods, like dairy, may be well tolerated, while fruit and wheat (baked goods) may not. What a treat to find the offenders while preserving the delights!*

### WHAT DO I NEED TO DO?

1. Check each symptom you are currently experiencing in the Disease/ Symptom Questionnaire below.

2. Grade the level of discomfort you have on a scale from 0–10 (with "0" being no symptom at all to a "10" being severe discomfort).

3. Be sure to check the symptoms and grade your level of discomfort AGAIN at the end of each Food Phase or every four weeks.

4. Take the results with you to your next medical appointment. Talk about how you're feeling and whether or not you still need any prescription medications for IBS.

### IBS Disease/Symptom Questionnaire

| Symptom Experience | Level of Discomfort | | |
|---|---|---|---|
| **Abdominal Pain (cramping, bloating, aching)** | None<br>0 1 2 3 4 5 6 7 | | Severe<br>8 9 10 |
| **Gas** | None<br>0 1 2 3 4 5 6 7 | | Severe<br>8 9 10 |
| **Diarrhea** | None<br>0 1 2 3 4 5 6 7 | | Severe<br>8 9 10 |
| **Constipation** | None<br>0 1 2 3 4 5 6 7 | | Severe<br>8 9 10 |

\* **WARNING: Never discontinue a prescribed medication without consulting with your healthcare provider.**

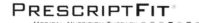

## PRESCRIPTFIT®
MEDICAL NUTRITION THERAPY ■ ■ ■ ■ ■ ■ ■

# ～ Section C: Getting Well... ～

## Sleep Apnea/Snoring

### What is Sleep Apnea?

Sleep apnea is a sleep disorder that affects some 18 million Americans and can be very serious if not treated. People with this disorder stop breathing for 10 to 30 seconds at a time while they are sleeping, possibly as many as 400 times each night. These periods of not breathing often wake you from deep sleep, seriously reducing the amount of necessary rest you actually get.

Those with sleep apnea typically suffer progressive fatigue, tiredness, malaise, depression, and muscle stiffness. Sleep apnea is associated with increased risk for heart attack and stroke. In addition, this common disorder can lead to disability and death from motor vehicle accidents that occur when the person falls asleep at the wheel from extreme tiredness.

Treatment typically involves use of dental devices, equipment that increases air pressure to increase restful breathing during sleep, and weight loss.

### What Causes Sleep Apnea?

"Obstructive" sleep apnea is what nine out of 10 people with sleep apnea have and is caused by something blocking the passage or windpipe (called the trachea) that brings air into your body. That something may be:

> Your tongue, tonsils, or the uvula (the small piece of flesh hanging down in the back of the throat).

> Excessive fatty tissue in the throat; many people with sleep apnea are obese.

*Snoring may be a key indicator of sleep apnea; it is common with aging and in those with sleep disorders.*

*Sleep disorders are studied in certified sleep laboratories available in most communities.*

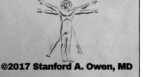

©2017 Stanford A. Owen, MD

**PRESCRIPTFIT**®
MEDICAL NUTRITION THERAPY ▪ ▪ ▪ ▪ ▪ ▪ ▪

# CHAPTER 9: FIRST-LINE TREATMENT

> Abnormally relaxed throat muscles, due to poor function of the nerves from the lower brain that control breathing and swallowing. Evidence suggest the poor nerve function is related to abnormal metabolism.

## WHAT ROLE MIGHT CYTOKINE IMBALANCE PLAY?

The exact role that cytokines have on sleep is unknown. Studies show that most sleep apnea patients have excess levels of cytokines associated with inflammation, which attach directly to nerve cells in the brain, including the areas that control breathing and swallowing.

*Diet can acutely affect your sleep, especially large fatty meals with excessive calories, carbohydrates, and alcohol.*

## WHAT RESULTS COULD I EXPECT WITH MNT?

MNT is the first line of treatment recommended in obese or overweight patients with sleep disorders. Patients using the Plan note improvement in fatigue by the end of Food Phases 1 and 2 of the 7- to 14-day Plans.

With MNT, many patients can eventually discontinue annoying and expensive sleep devices. Nutritional diets appear to be far more important than weight loss in treating sleep apnea. In most patients, improvement in fatigue and snoring diminishes long before large weight loss is noted. In fact, patients who undergo gastric bypass operations often can stop using special breathing devices for sleep apnea within weeks — long before they experience significant weight loss.

## HOW CAN I MEASURE SYMPTOM CHANGE ON THE PLAN?

First, you need to be clear about what may be causing your sleep apnea. Although rare, there is a second type of sleep apnea (central sleep apnea) that occurs when the muscles you use to

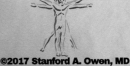

**PRESCRIPTFIT**
MEDICAL NUTRITION THERAPY ▪ ▪ ▪ ▪ ▪ ▪ ▪

breathe fail for some reason to receive the signal to do so from your brain. You should work with your healthcare provider to clearly identify which type of sleep apnea you have and what would be the best treatment approach. Talk with your healthcare provider about the effects that MNT may have on your treatment. Next, you want to measure how severe each of the two, key sleep apnea symptoms are for you. This will give you a "baseline" to compare with future measurements.

Most importantly, you (and your provider) need a way to measure progress over time. Talk with your healthcare provider at each regular visit about your symptoms and how they might change using the Plan.

## WHAT DO I NEED TO DO?

1. *Check your level of energy and snoring in the Disease/Symptom Questionnaire below. For snoring, your partner may be more knowledgeable about your symptoms than you are.*

2. *Grade the level of discomfort you have on a scale from 0–10 (with "0" being normal energy and no snoring, respectively, and "10" being no energy and severe snoring, respectively).*

3. *Be sure to check the symptoms and grade your level of discomfort AGAIN at the end of each Food Phase or every four weeks.*

4. *Take the results with you to your next medical appointment. Talk about how you're feeling and whether or not you still need conventional treatments for sleep apnea.*

### SLEEP APNEA DISEASE/SYMPTOM QUESTIONNAIRE

| Symptom Experience | Level of Discomfort | | |
|---|---|---|---|
| **Fatigue/Energy Level** | **Normal Energy** | | **No Energy** |
| | 0 1 2 3 4 5 6 7 8 9 10 | | |
| **Snoring** | **None** | | **Severe** |
| | 0 1 2 3 4 5 6 7 8 9 10 | | |

* **WARNING: Never discontinue a prescribed medication without consulting with your healthcare provider.**

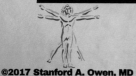

©2017 Stanford A. Owen, MD

PRESCRIPTFIT®
MEDICAL NUTRITION THERAPY ▪ ▪ ▪ ▪ ▪ ▪ ▪ ▪

# CHAPTER 9: FIRST-LINE TREATMENT

## STEATOSIS (FATTY LIVER)

### WHAT IS STEATOSIS?

Steatosis or "fatty liver" is the most common form of chronic liver disease, replacing alcohol and viral hepatitis as the most common cause of cirrhosis of the liver. Patients with fatty liver and alcoholism or viral hepatitis are much more likely to have liver cell damage and cirrhosis.

### WHAT CAUSES FATTY LIVER?

Fatty liver is caused by the accumulation of triglyceride fat deposits within liver cells due to abnormal liver metabolism. Excessive fat in liver cells provokes inflammation and activates the immune system. Simple blood tests can suggest the presence of inflammation caused by these fat deposits but cannot assure the definitive cause.

Because the only way to prove a diagnosis of steatosis is to perform a biopsy of the liver (which carries a risk of bleeding), many physicians make the diagnosis by exclusion. That is, for those who have NEITHER a history of alcoholism nor lab results indicating a viral/immune liver disease, there is a 90 percent chance that your symptoms indicate a fatty liver — odds reasonable enough to avoid biopsy.

*If your healthcare provider finds that your lab tests do not improve or normalize when you carefully follow the Plan, a biopsy may be required.*

### WHAT ROLE MIGHT CYTOKINE IMBALANCE PLAY?

Most patients with fatty liver are overweight. Patients with fatty liver have elevated levels of inflammation cytokines (CRP, IL-6, TNF). Patients with fatty liver often have diabetes or pre-diabetes (IRS), conditions also associated with abnormal cytokine production. Studies suggest the fat accumulation and the inflammation of the liver cell

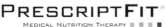

*People with fatty liver tend to be more likely to suffer with metabolic syndrome (insulin resistant syndrome) and eventually be diagnosed with diabetes. They have a higher rate of hypertension and sleep apnea as well as elevated cholesterol and triglyceride levels.*

are related but independent abnormalities. Common cytokines may play a role in both, and nutrition may be the common mediator.

### What Results Could I Expect with MNT?

MNT is the first line of treatment for fatty liver, especially because of the Plan's ability to help you reduce your triglyceride levels. Patients using the Plan improve laboratory tests of fatty liver usually by the end of Food Phase 8 of the 7-day or Food Phase 4 of the 14-day Plan. Your healthcare provider should perform liver function tests (SGOT, SGPT, and alkaline phosphatase blood tests) every 12 weeks when using the Plan.

### How Can I Measure Symptom Change on the Plan?

Improvement in fatty liver enzyme results must be measured by your healthcare provider. Share the Disease/Symptom Questionnaire below with your provider; measurement should be considered every 12 weeks until your lab results indicate that the maximum response has been achieved.

| STEATOSIS (FATTY LIVER) DISEASE/SYMPTOM QUESTIONNAIRE | |
|---|---|
| **INITIAL LAB VALUES** | **12-WEEK LAB VALUES** |
| SGOT _____ | SGOT _____ |
| SGPT _____ | SGPT _____ |
| ALKALINE PHOSPHATASE _____ | ALKALINE PHOSPHATASE _____ |

**\* WARNING: Never discontinue a prescribed medication without consulting with your healthcare provider.**

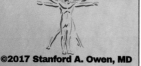

PRESCRIPTFIT
MEDICAL NUTRITION THERAPY ■ ■ ■ ■ ■ ■ ■

## CHAPTER 10: ENHANCING WELLNESS WITH MNT

The Plan is designed to help you discover for yourself how to craft your most successful lifestyle by letting you learn what works and what doesn't at each step of nutrition change. You will probably experience some remission (absence or significant reduction of troublesome symptoms) as well as relapse (a return to illness). Because PrescriptFit measures outcome, you quickly learn how and where to adjust your plan away from danger and toward health.

**MNT can be used to assist treatment for a number of illnesses and chronic conditions, such as:**

> Angina Pectoris
> Asthma
> Back Pain
> Congestive Heart Failure
> Depression
> Dyspnea (Breathlessness)
> Edema (Swelling)
> Fatigue
> Fibromyalgia
> Infertility
> Insomnia
> Joint Pain

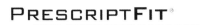

PRESCRIPTFIT®
MEDICAL NUTRITION THERAPY ▪ ▪ ▪ ▪ ▪ ▪ ▪ ▪

## ANGINA PECTORIS
## (CHEST PAIN, HEART PAIN, CHEST PRESSURE, CHEST HEAVINESS)

### WHAT IS ANGINA PECTORIS?

*Half of all heart attack victims die prior to reaching medical care; yet most experienced warning symptoms.*

Angina is described as pain, pressure, crushing, pressing, heavy, or breathless discomfort in the chest. Angina may radiate to the back, neck, or down the arms. It may be mild to severe.

Angina may be precipitated by exertion, emotion, food, smoking, sleeplessness, altitude, and other factors that alter the tone of small blood vessels. It is often worse in the morning.

*Any angina symptoms (not previously diagnosed by a healthcare provider) warrant immediate attention.*

Angina can be both disabling and frightening. Usually present prior to a heart attack, angina is often ignored as "indigestion" or associated with fatigue and exhaustion (especially in women).

### WHAT CAUSES ANGINA PECTORIS?

Angina pain originates from the heart, caused by insufficient blood flow through the arteries caused by spasm or cholesterol blockage of the coronary arteries.

### WHAT ROLE MIGHT CYTOKINE IMBALANCE PLAY?

Small blood vessels react to changes in excess calories, sugar, and fat. Improvement in blood vessel function improves using branched-chain amino acids. Cytokines have direct influence on small vessel lining to cause spasm, increase clotting, and damage collagen that keeps the vessel supple and pliable.

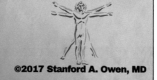

**PRESCRIPTFIT**
MEDICAL NUTRITION THERAPY ▪ ▪ ▪ ▪ ▪ ▪ ▪

# ⌁ CHAPTER 10: ENHANCING WELLNESS ⌁

## WHAT RESULTS COULD I EXPECT WITH MNT?

Those using the Plan often note immediate and substantial relief of angina, especially in Food Phases 1 and 2. Likewise, patients may experience immediate pain relapse even after a large meal, especially if high in fat and sugar.

Angina may be very sensitive to amount of food, type of food, and even preparation of food (as with use of fatty condiments). Remain alert to improvement and relapse of symptoms.

## HOW CAN I MEASURE SYMPTOM CHANGE ON THE PLAN?

Angina can be sporadic or predictable. If your experience with angina is predictable, you will find improvement the easiest to measure. For example, you may feel angina every time you walk to the mailbox up the hill and have to rest or take a nitroglycerine tablet to resolve the discomfort. Being able to complete the walk without stopping would be a measurable improvement you could readily see. If your experience with angina is more sporadic, it may take some time to see a trend that indicates less episodes of discomfort.

First, you need to make sure that you see your healthcare provider immediately for any symptoms of angina that have not been previously diagnosed. Your provider will prescribe treatment after determining what course of cardiac care is best for you. You will need to follow that treatment carefully. MNT can support your treatment plan with the combined benefits of branched-chain amino acids and how you monitor changes throughout the Food Phases.

Next, you want to have a measurement of how frequent, severe, and long lasting each episode of angina is for you. This will give you a "baseline" to compare with future measurements.

*Important: You (and your healthcare provider) need a way to measure progress over time. Talk with your provider at each visit about your symptoms and how they might change using the Plan.*

**PRESCRIPTFIT**®
MEDICAL NUTRITION THERAPY ▪ ▪ ▪ ▪ ▪ ▪ ▪

# SECTION C: GETTING WELL...

Of medications prescribed to reduce symptoms, nitroglycerin is perhaps the best known. However, you should record whether or not you take this medication and if it offers relief during the episodes you measure. Also record the same information for other medications your healthcare provider may prescribe for this condition.

## WHAT DO I NEED TO DO?

1. *Determine how often you experience angina in the Disease/Symptom Questionnaire below.*

2. *Grade the level of discomfort you have as well as the duration of the discomfort on the Questionnaire as indicated.*

3. *Indicate whether or not nitroglycerin relieved the discomfort as well as other medications prescribed.*

4. *Be sure to grade your angina episodes AGAIN at the end of each Food Phase or every four weeks.*

5. *Take the results with you to your next medical appointment. Talk about how you're feeling and whether or not you still need any prescription medications for angina.*

6. *If symptoms relapse, return to the previous Phase and progress again. If angina returns with the same Food Phase each time, eliminate the provoking food. When returning to prior Phases, progress through each one more slowly to clearly identify the offending food group.*

## ANGINA PECTORIS DISEASE/SYMPTOM QUESTIONNAIRE

### Angina Discomfort

| | | | |
|---|---|---|---|
| **Frequency** | ❑ **Daily** | ❑ **<3/Day** | ❑ **≥3/Day** |
| **Intensity (average)** | ❑ **Mild** | ❑ **Moderate** | ❑ **Severe** |
| **Duration** | ❑ **≤1 minute** | ❑ **≤5 minutes** | ❑ **≤30 minutes** |

### Relief from Medications

| | | |
|---|---|---|
| **Nitroglycerin** | ❑ **YES** | ❑ **No** |
| **Other Medication** (angina prevention or treatment) | ❑ **YES** | ❑ **No** |

\* **WARNING: Never discontinue a prescribed medication without consulting with your healthcare provider.**

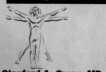

**PRESCRIPTFIT**
MEDICAL NUTRITION THERAPY ▪ ▪ ▪ ▪ ▪ ▪ ▪

# ⌐ CHAPTER 10: ENHANCING WELLNESS ⌐

## ASTHMA

### WHAT IS ASTHMA?

Asthma is a chronic lung disease that affects nearly 20 million people in the U.S. People with asthma typically experience spontaneous episodes of difficult breathing. These result from inflammation in the lungs that causes airways to become blocked or narrowed. When this happens, the lungs also produce more mucus, which further hinders breathing and may cause wheezing and coughing. People with asthma may suffer more at night or in early morning.

*The incidence of asthma is increased markedly in the obese (both children and adults). The epidemic increase of asthma in children that has occurred in the last two decades may be, in part, related to the epidemic of childhood obesity.*

### WHAT CAUSES ASTHMA?

Asthma can be caused by an allergic reaction or triggered by a number of factors not related to allergies, such as being exposed to cold air, exercise, or having heartburn (reflux). Although there is no single, known cause, environmental factors (e.g., tobacco smoke, pollutants, stress) or biological ones — related to one's internal chemistry (e.g., food or drug allergies) — appear to trigger attacks.

The main contributor to asthma is inflammation within the lungs leading to constriction of the airway muscles, stimulation of mucous production, and flooding of the airways with inflammatory cells.

### WHAT ROLE MIGHT CYTOKINE IMBALANCE PLAY?

Because cytokines trigger inflammation that may result in asthma, branched-chain amino acids' ability to reduce out-of-balance cytokines can significantly help reduce symptoms. Most new asthma medications directly attack cytokines (called leukotrienes). Therefore, logic dictates a trial of MNT to measure asthma improvement.

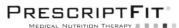

**PRESCRIPTFIT**
MEDICAL NUTRITION THERAPY ▪ ▪ ▪ ▪ ▪ ▪ ▪

# ～ Section C: Getting Well... ～

*The beauty of the Food Phase Plan is your ability to carefully add in each food group and isolate exactly which foods might trigger asthma attacks. .*

## What Results Could I Expect with MNT?

Based on clinical data, asthma improves in many patients using the MNT Plan, especially in Food Phases 1 and 2. Additionally, PrescriptFit may improve asthma by removing the thousands of different nutrients, bacteria, and chemicals in a normal diet. Food Phases 1 and 2 of the Plan limit exposure to nutrients and particles that might trigger inflammation. As a specific food group is added in, note if asthma worsens. A specific food group may contribute to asthma in one person but not another. Those foods high in fat, sugar, and dairy products should be especially monitored to see if symptoms worsen after eating.

## How Can I Measure Symptom Change on the Plan?

First, see your healthcare provider right away for any symptoms of asthma. Have him or her share with you what measurements indicate that you have asthma and if your asthma might be from an allergy. Next, complete the Disease/Symptom Questionnaire at right for a "baseline" to compare with future measures.

*Note that some measurements associated with monitoring asthma must be done in a health care setting, especially measurements of lung flow (referred to as the "Peak Flow" test). Peak Flow "meters" are available at any drugstore and are recommended for asthma patients home use.*

Most importantly, you (and your provider) need a way to measure progress over time. Talk with your healthcare provider at each regular visit about your symptoms and how they might change using the Plan. Be sure to have your healthcare provider take the same measurements after 12 weeks on the MNT Plan as you had taken at the "baseline" mark.

With PrescriptFit, you may find that as your symptoms lessen, you will need to take less medication OR perhaps discontinue your medications entirely. If you are taking prescription medicines, talk to your healthcare provider about when and how to cut down on what you take BEFORE you make any changes.

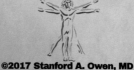

# PrescriptFit®
MEDICAL NUTRITION THERAPY ■ ■ ■ ■ ■ ■ ■

# ⟶ CHAPTER 10: ENHANCING WELLNESS ⟶

## WHAT DO I NEED TO DO?

1. See your healthcare provider to determine if you have asthma and whether or not an allergy might be related to your symptoms. Have the healthcare provider take a baseline measurement of lung flow and record the results.
2. Use the Disease/Symptom Questionnaire below to record:
   - Your level of discomfort/severity using the on a scale of 0–10 ("0" indicates mild symptoms and "10" indicates the most severe problems). Re-measure asthma symptoms after each Food Phase of the Plan.
   - The type of inhaler and frequency of use and other prescribed medications
   - How fast and how completely symptoms resolve. (When symptoms relapse, note which Food Phase you're in, return to the one before, and progress again. Also note relapse that occurs at the same Phase each time.)
3. Have your provider measure lung flow 12 weeks after beginning the Plan.
4. Review results with your provider; ask how your medication needs may change as your symptoms change.

### ASTHMA DISEASE/SYMPTOM QUESTIONNAIRE

| Symptom | Level of Discomfort | | |
|---|---|---|---|
| **Breathlessness** | Mild | Moderate | Severe |
| | 0  1  2  3 | 4  5  6  7 | 8  9  10 |
| **Coughing** | Infrequent | Frequent | Constant |
| | 0  1  2  3 | 4  5  6  7 | 8  9  10 |
| **Wheezing** | Occasional | Often | Constant |
| | 0  1  2  3 | 4  5  6  7 | 8  9  10 |
| **Sputum Production** | None/Minimal | Moderate | Constant |
| | 0  1  2  3 | 4  5  6  7 | 8  9  10 |
| **Impact on Quality of Life** | None Nuisance Interferes Alters Threatens | | |
| | 0  1  2  3  4  5  6  7  8  9  10 | | |

**Lung Flow Measure (medical testing): Peak Flow _____ liters/minute**

**Inhalers**

| Frequency of Use # puffs/day: ☐1 ☐2 ☐3 ☐4 ☐>4 # days/week: ☐1 ☐2 ☐3 ☐4 ☐>4 | Number Used (check those used and total) ☐ Albuterol /Salbuterol   ☐ Steroid Inhaler ☐ Atrovent   ☐ Chromalyn ☐ Combination Inhalers (Combivent™, Advair™) Total _____ |
|---|---|

**Oral Medications:** ☐ Theophylline      ☐ Brethine

\* WARNING: Never discontinue prescribed medication without consulting with a healthcare provider.

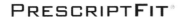

**PRESCRIPTFIT**®
MEDICAL NUTRITION THERAPY ▪ ▪ ▪ ▪ ▪ ▪ ▪          ©2017 Stanford A. Owen, MD

## BACK PAIN

### WHAT IS BACK PAIN?

Back pain is an ongoing aching, soreness, and/ or strained feeling in the back anywhere from the shoulders to the hips. It occurs in everyone at some point in life. It can result from some acute injury as well as chronic strain from poor posture, excessive weight, or both. Some health conditions, such as kidney infection, can cause severe pain and soreness in the mid portion of the back. You should always consult with your healthcare provider about any unexplained back pain to be sure that you are not suffering from some illness that requires immediate treatment.

*Back pain is present in almost every obese person.*

### WHAT CAUSES BACK PAIN?

For chronic back pain that results from ongoing strain due to weight, cause is related to your body's attempts to adjust your form to your changing body shape. As weight increases, abdominal size expands forward, causing stress along the ligaments and muscles connecting the vertebrae and collagen discs; the result — chronic pain.

### WHAT ROLE MIGHT CYTOKINE IMBALANCE PLAY?

There is evidence that cytokines produced by fat cells may lead to direct injury of collagen, weakening the ligaments, tendons, and spinal discs. Fat cells also produce inflaming cytokine proteins that may damage the lining of joints, including the small joints separating each vertebrae that allow you to easily bend, twist, and stretch the spine.

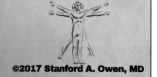

PRESCRIPTFIT®
MEDICAL NUTRITION THERAPY ▪ ▪ ▪ ▪ ▪ ▪ ▪

# CHAPTER 10: ENHANCING WELLNESS

## WHAT RESULTS COULD I EXPECT WITH MNT?

The MNT Plan will reduce the excessive weight and cytokines that contribute to back strain. Based on over a decade of clinical experience, 67 percent of patients who visit our clinic can discontinue medication for back pain within six months after they begin using the MNT Plan combined with physical therapy or rehabilitative exercise. For those taking anti-inflammatory medications for back pain, there's an added bonus of stomach complaints improving — both from the reduced need to take the anti-inflammatory medications AND from eliminating irritating foods using the MNT Food Phase approach to identify those causing digestive problems.

## HOW CAN I MEASURE SYMPTOM CHANGE ON THE PLAN?

First, you need to be clear about what is causing your back pain. If you're overweight, work in a job that requires lifting and other strenuous activities, or have recently strained your back, you should talk to your healthcare provider about the benefits of the MNT Plan as well as physical therapy/rehabilitative exercise. If your back pain has occurred recently without explanation or apparent cause, your provider will need to determine if there might be a more serious illness causing your discomfort that requires treatment.

Next, you want to have a measurement of how severe your back pain is on a daily basis. This will give you a "baseline" to compare with future measurements.

Most importantly, you (and your provider) need a way to measure progress over time. Talk with your provider at each regular visit about your symptoms and how they have changed using the Plan.

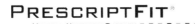

PRESCRIPTFIT
MEDICAL NUTRITION THERAPY

# ⁓ Section C: Getting Well... ⁓

As with any medical condition, treatment traditionally means taking medications to reduce symptoms. A number of prescription and over-the-counter medications can be taken to reduce the pain and inflammation in your back. With MNT, you may find that you will need to take less medication OR perhaps discontinue your medications entirely. If you are taking prescription medicines, talk to your healthcare provider about when and how to cut down on what you take BEFORE you make any changes.

## WHAT DO I NEED TO DO?

1. Grade the level of daily discomfort you have on a scale from 0–10 (with "0" being mild and "10" being severe discomfort).

2. Be sure to grade your level of discomfort AGAIN at the end of each Food Phase or every four weeks.

3. Record the number of medications you currently take for back pain. Be sure to record how many pain medications you're taking at the end of each Food Phase or every four weeks.

4. Take the results with you to your next medical appointment. Talk about how you're feeling and whether or not you still need medications for back pain.

### BACK PAIN DISEASE/SYMPTOM QUESTIONNAIRE

| Average Daily Back Pain | Mild Moderate Severe 0 1 2 3 4 5 6 7 8 9 10 |
|---|---|
| **Number of medications taken daily** _____ **(e.g., aspirin + Tylenol = 2 medications)** | |

\* WARNING: Never discontinue a prescribed medication without consulting with your healthcare provider.

PRESCRIPTFIT
MEDICAL NUTRITION THERAPY ▪ ▪ ▪ ▪ ▪ ▪ ▪

# ᗗ CHAPTER 10: ENHANCING WELLNESS ᗒ

## CONGESTIVE HEART FAILURE (CHF)

### WHAT IS CONGESTIVE HEART FAILURE (CHF)?

Congestive Heart Failure occurs when the heart can't pump enough blood to supply the body's organs. "Back-pressure" of blood leads to lung congestion, producing breathlessness and shortness of breath. The kidney has more trouble getting rid of sodium and water when blood flow is compromised, which results in swelling (edema) of the legs.

Patients with CHF struggle to breathe when walking, wake up at night breathless, and "give out" easily.

Patients with CHF often demonstrate dramatic improvement using the Prescript Fit™ MNT Plan. MNT could be an integral part of CHF treatment since type and amount of nutrients affect fluid retention.

*Patients with CHF should use PrescriptFit MNT Plan only under direct and close medical supervision.*

### WHAT CAUSES CHF?

Age and obesity are the two major causes of CHF. As heart tissue ages, it has more trouble pumping blood with the same efficiency of a "younger" heart. Similarly, the heart must pump substantially harder when one is obese. CHF can also result from heart muscle damage after a heart attack, prolonged uncontrolled high blood pressure, and malfunctioning heart valves. Nutritional deficiency further weakens heart muscle cells.

Cytokines play a dominant role in CHF via fluid balance, excess clotting, repair and renewal of injured heart cells, and small blood vessel malfunction. The dramatic improvement seen in CHF patients (under medical guidance) with

*Diabetes, in particular, can directly cause CHF by injuring heart muscle through poor metabolism of nutrients and toxic damage from cytokines. Patients with diabetes who also suffer from CHF often improve with MNT.*

PRESCRIPTFIT
MEDICAL NUTRITION THERAPY ▪ ▪ ▪ ▪ ▪ ▪ ▪ ▪

# ≈ Section C: Getting Well... ≈

MNT may be, in part, due to balancing of cytokine function. Excess fluid is removed, blood vessels relax, clotting diminishes, and heart cells function better. Scarring of the heart lessens.

## What Results Could I Expect with MNT?

In our clinic, improvement with MNT has been unrelated to amount of weight loss. Certainly, decreased weight equals decreased stress on the heart. However, the percentage improvement noted typically occurs within the first 12 weeks of starting MNT, usually in the first two weeks — long before meaningful fat loss occurs. Patients who comply with PrescriptFit maintenance strategies following all Food Phases can often diminish fluid medication with medical guidance. **CHF patients should keep in close contact with their healthcare providers during Food Phase 1. Do not regulate medication on your own.**

Use the 14-day Plan to clearly determine which food groups or what quantity of food will cause fluid retention. While difficult to follow, the improvement usually far outweighs the deprivation. Even a 7-day/ Phase strategy provides significant improvement in most cases.

## How Can I Measure Symptom Change on the Plan?

First, you need to be clear about what might be causing your symptoms of CHF. Visit your healthcare provider to determine if edema or shortness of breath could stem from some other illness. Next, you want to have a measurement of how severe each symptom is for you. This will give you a "baseline" to compare with future measurements.

*Patients with CHF can lose 20–50 pounds of fluid in Food Phases 1 and 2, demonstrating the powerful effect of dietary influences on cardiovascular physiology.*

*Tell your healthcare provider about the review available in the American Journal of Cardiology Supplement, April 2004: "The Role of Nutritional Supplements with Essential Amino Acids in Patients with Cardiovascular Disease and Diabetes Mellitus."*

**PRESCRIPTFIT**
MEDICAL NUTRITION THERAPY ▪ ▪ ▪ ▪ ▪ ▪ ▪

# ⌁ CHAPTER 10: ENHANCING WELLNESS ⌁

Most importantly, you (and your provider) need a way to measure progress over time. Talk with your healthcare provider at each visit about your symptoms and how they might change using the PrescriptFit Plan.

As with any medical condition, treatment traditionally means taking medications to reduce symptoms. With PrescriptFit, you may find that as your symptoms lessen, you will need to take less medication OR perhaps discontinue your medications entirely.

*If you are taking prescription medicines, talk to your healthcare provider about when and how to cut down on what you take BEFORE you make any changes.*

## WHAT DO I NEED TO DO?

1. *Check each symptom you are currently experiencing in the Disease/ Symptom Questionnaire below.*
2. *Grade the level of discomfort you have on a scale from 0–10 (with "0" being no symptom or problem and "10" being severe discomfort or lack of stamina).*
3. *Be sure to check the symptoms and grade your level of discomfort AGAIN at the end of each Food Phase or every four weeks.*
4. *Take the results with you to your next medical appointment. Talk about how you're feeling and what changes you might be able to make to your prescribed medications for CHF.*

### CONGESTIVE HEART FAILURE
### DISEASE/SYMPTOM QUESTIONNAIRE

| Symptom Experience | Level of Discomfort |
|---|---|
| **Edema/Fluid Retention** | **None**        **Severe**<br>0 1 2 3 4 5 6 7 8 9 10 |
| **Shortness of Breath** | **None**        **Severe**<br>0 1 2 3 4 5 6 7 8 9 10 |
| **Orthopnea (Inability to breathe easily when lying flat)** | **No Problem**      **Severe**<br>0 1 2 3 4 5 6 7 8 9 10 |
| **Stamina/Sense of Well Being** | **Normal**      **No Stamina**<br>0 1 2 3 4 5 6 7 8 9 10 |

\* WARNING: Never discontinue a prescribed medication without consulting with your healthcare provider.

## PRESCRIPTFIT®
MEDICAL NUTRITION THERAPY ▪ ▪ ▪ ▪ ▪ ▪ ▪

## SECTION C: GETTING WELL...

## DEPRESSION

### WHAT IS DEPRESSION?

Depression is a chronic psychiatric condition that can be very debilitating or even life threatening. People who are depressed will typically feel sad and hopeless, may have changes in eating and sleeping patterns, and may move and think more slowly than usual. If severe, they may think about or plan suicide. The most common symptoms include being fatigued and unmotivated to participate in or enjoy activities that used to be pleasurable (including sex).

### WHAT CAUSES DEPRESSION?

We don't know exactly what causes depression; however, experts agree that some people are more prone to depression than others and that certain events or situations can put these people at risk for suffering from the illness. What we do know is that there are chemicals in the brain that impact how we handle stress, and these chemicals appear to be out of balance for those diagnosed with depression.

Many medical conditions and some medications can contribute to symptoms of depression. People with depression often struggle with anxiety or mood swings as well. In addition, poor nutrition may contribute to depression. People who are depressed often either eat too much because it's soothing or eat too little because they have no appetite or energy for eating. Nutritional balance certainly suffers either way.

*See your healthcare provider about any depression symptoms lasting more than two weeks; a thorough evaluation by a healthcare provider experienced in treating depression is very important for arriving at the right diagnosis and getting optimal therapy.*

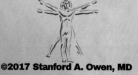

©2017 Stanford A. Owen, MD

## PRESCRIPTFIT
MEDICAL NUTRITION THERAPY ■ ■ ■ ■ ■ ■ ■

# CHAPTER 10: ENHANCING WELLNESS

## WHAT ROLE MIGHT CYTOKINE IMBALANCE PLAY?

Brain chemicals (called neurotransmitters) are intimately influenced by cytokines produced by fat, liver, and immune tissues. Depression is more common, for instance, in patients who overproduce C-Reactive Protein (or CRP) — common in those with metabolic syndrome, heart disease, and diabetes. Other cytokines called "interleukins" (IL-6, IL-2, and others) are closely tied to depression. The most dramatic example is the adverse side effect experienced by some when taking interferon (related to interleukin). Interferon is used for treating viral hepatitis; the profound depression that results in many cases often requires discontinuing the treatment.

Other cytokine hormones (leptin, ghrelin, cholecystokinin) have dramatic effects on eating behavior, which in turn, may lead to metabolic problems that contribute to depression.

The brain's nerve cells have receptors that are very sensitive to changes in cytokine production, nutrition balance, and external factors. The common receptors known to affect depression (serotonin, dopamine, and norepinephrine) are also intricately tied to energy metabolism. Most antidepressants cause weight gain by impacting how these neurochemicals affect eating behavior and energy expenditure (exercise and activity). Many of these antidepressants also raise cytokine levels, occasionally dramatically, and can even cause or precipitate diabetes.

*These facts alone make a strong case for cytokine and brain happiness being connected. The future holds great promise for improved depression treatment and improved metabolism as we unravel these delicate chemical interactions.*

## WHAT RESULTS COULD I EXPECT WITH MNT?

The symptoms of depression most likely to improve with MNT are fatigue (lack of energy), joy, motivation, and sex drive. Based on over a decade of clinical experience, these symptoms

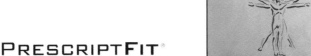

**PRESCRIPTFIT**®
MEDICAL NUTRITION THERAPY ▪ ▪ ▪ ▪ ▪ ▪ ▪

©2017 Stanford A. Owen, MD

# SECTION C: GETTING WELL...

most dramatically improve during Food Phase 1 of the Plan.

Because some antidepressant medications may contribute to weight gain and sexual dysfunction, it's important to talk to your healthcare provider about how possible medication side effects might impact your general health. MNT may play a vital role in managing side effects that could occur with those medications that may best treat your depressive symptoms.

At the very least, PrescriptFit offers balanced nutrition for balanced brain function while reducing the levels of toxic cytokines known to be associated with depression. A lower, leaner weight will improve self confidence, make movement (exercise) easier, and will gain more favorable social interaction from others — factors all known to effect depression.

### HOW CAN I MEASURE SYMPTOM CHANGE WITH THE PLAN?

First, visit your healthcare provider to determine what might be causing your depression. Next, score the DOCTORdiet Psychological Profile (online at www.drdiet.com) prior to starting the Plan, and rate your level of hopelessness in the Disease/Symptom Questionnaire on the next page. This will give you a baseline measurement of how depressed you feel.

Most importantly, you (and your provider) need a way to measure progress over time. Take the DOCTORdiet Psychological Profile again after Food Phase 1, and after 12 weeks (for those following the 7- or 14-day Plan). Re-score yourself every 12 weeks thereafter. Discuss with your provider at each regular visit how your symptoms might change using the PrescriptFit Plan.

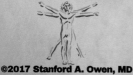

**PRESCRIPTFIT**®
MEDICAL NUTRITION THERAPY ▪ ▪ ▪ ▪ ▪ ▪ ▪

# ⌐ CHAPTER 10: ENHANCING WELLNESS ⌐

As you progress through the Plan, note how you feel when adding each food category. If a particular food seems to be related to when you experience symptoms of depression, share this information with your healthcare provider and use the knowledge you gain to modify your diet.

As with any medical condition, treatment may involve taking medications to reduce your depression symptoms. Many of these medications require close medical supervision to change the dose or stop taking them. With PrescriptFit, you may find that as your symptoms lessen, you will need to take less medication OR perhaps discontinue your medications entirely.

*Do not change how often or how much of your prescription medication you take without medical approval; serious side effects or complications could result.*

## WHAT DO I NEED TO DO?

1. *See your healthcare provider to determine what might be causing your symptoms. Talk with your provider about incorporating MNT into your treatment plan.*

2. *Take the DOCTORdiet Psychological Profile before beginning the PrescriptFit Plan. Take the Profile again after Food Phase I and after 12 weeks on the Plan.*

3. *Record your symptoms of depression on the Disease/Symptom Questionnaire below on a scale of 0–10 with "0" being "none" and "10" being "thoughts of suicide." Be sure to record your discomfort level again at the end of each Food Phase or every four weeks.*

4. *Review the results with your healthcare provider —talk about how you're feeling and changes in your need for prescription medications and doses prescribed based on MNT results.*

## DEPRESSION DISEASE/SYMPTOM QUESTIONNAIRE

| Depression Rating* | None | | | | | | | | | Thoughts of Suicide |
|---|---|---|---|---|---|---|---|---|---|---|
| | 0 1 2 3 4 5 6 7 8 9 10 | | | | | | | | | |

\* Complete the DOCTORdiet Psychological Profile (online at www.drdiet.com) as directed; NEVER alter how you take medications for depression without consulting your healthcare provider.

# PRESCRIPTFIT®
MEDICAL NUTRITION THERAPY ▪ ▪ ▪ ▪ ▪ ▪ ▪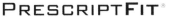

©2017 Stanford A. Owen, MD

# DYSPNEA (BREATHLESSNESS)

### WHAT IS DYSPNEA?

*You should see your healthcare provider if you have any symptoms of breathlessness.*

Dyspnea, or breathlessness, is any perceived difficulty breathing or pain you feel when breathing. It can be a symptom of many disorders, especially:

> Cardiac disease (coronary obstruction, CHF, valve disease, other)

> Pulmonary disease (asthma, emphysema, other)

> Kidney disease with edema (swelling)

> Liver disease with edema (swelling)

> Anemia (iron deficiency, B-12 deficiency, other)

> Hypothyroidism

### WHAT CAUSES DYSPNEA?

Breathlessness may be caused by medical conditions or simply by excessive weight. Breathlessness may be a symptom of underlying cardiac disease. Healthcare provider evaluation is recommended, including a cardiac stress test and cardiac ultrasound exam. A chest x-ray is also indicated, especially in smokers.

If breathlessness resolves during Food Phase 1 or 2, cardiac causes are still possible. One would not expect breathlessness from excess weight to improve within 4 weeks of treatment, as only a minimal amount of weight would be lost relative to total needed to lose.

PRESCRIPTFIT®
MEDICAL NUTRITION THERAPY ▪ ▪ ▪ ▪ ▪ ▪

# ᴄCHAPTER 10: ENHANCING WELLNESS ᴄ

## WHAT ROLE MIGHT CYTOKINE IMBALANCE PLAY?

Cytokines are intimately involved with the function of small blood vessels and inflammation. Most of the conditions cited on the previous page have small blood vessel malfunction and/or inflammation as a primary component of the illness. While dyspnea is a symptom, it is related to cardiopulmonary function. Relaxing of the pulmonary (lung) small blood vessels and the small blood vessels downstream from the heart improve circulation, improve oxygen exchange, and therefore, improve dyspnea or breathlessness.

## WHAT RESULTS COULD I EXPECT WITH MNT?

Dyspnea improves very rapidly, in most cases, regardless of the primary cause (with the exception of emphysema). Most symptoms are measurably better in the first week. It's very reinforcing to track your ability to breathe better after each Plan phase. At the very least, improvement should be noted within four weeks. Breathlessness beyond this point is usually not improved by MNT.

Occasionally, a specific food may precipitate fluid retention, blood vessel spasm, or bronchial spasm leading to relapse of breathlessness. If breathlessness recurs when adding any specific food group, restart Food Phase 1 (with healthcare provider notification and supervision) and continue until symptoms resolve. Add the subsequent Food Phases slowly (every one to two weeks) and cautiously.

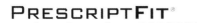

## ～ SECTION C: GETTING WELL... ～

### HOW CAN I MEASURE SYMPTOM CHANGE ON THE PLAN?

First, visit your healthcare provider to determine the cause of your breathlessness. Next, take a baseline measurement of the degree of discomfort you feel. Most importantly, you (and your healthcare provider) need a way to measure progress over time. Talk with your provider at each regular visit about your symptoms and how they might change using the Plan.

As with any medical condition, treatment may mean that you are taking medications to reduce your dyspnea symptoms. With this Plan, you may find that as your symptoms lessen, you will need to take less medication OR perhaps discontinue your medications entirely. If you are taking prescription medicines, talk to your healthcare provider about when and how to cut down on what you take BEFORE you make any changes.

### WHAT DO I NEED TO DO?

1. See your healthcare provider to determine what might be causing your symptoms. Talk with your healthcare provider about incorporating MNT into your treatment plan, depending on what medical condition might be causing the symptoms.

2. Record your level of discomfort on the Disease/Symptom Questionnaire below on a scale of 0–10 with "0" being "never breathless" and "10" being "always breathless." Be sure to record your discomfort level again at the end of each Food Phase or every four weeks.

3. Review the results with your healthcare provider — talk about how you're feeling and changes in your need for prescription medications and doses prescribed based on MNT results.

### DYSPNEA (BREATHLESSNESS) DISEASE/SYMPTOM QUESTIONNAIRE

| Frequency of Breathlessness | Never | | | | | | | | | | Always |
|---|---|---|---|---|---|---|---|---|---|---|---|
| | 0 | 1 | 2 | 3 | 4 | 5 | 6 | 7 | 8 | 9 | 10 |

\* WARNING: Do not discontinue or alter prescribed medications without first consulting with your healthcare provider.

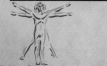

**PRESCRIPTFIT**®
MEDICAL NUTRITION THERAPY ■ ■ ■ ■ ■ ■ ■

# ⌁ CHAPTER 10: ENHANCING WELLNESS ⌁

## EDEMA (SWELLING)

### WHAT IS EDEMA?

Edema is visible swelling in the body, especially the feet and legs. This swelling occurs as a result of excess fluid accumulating under the skin in the spaces around blood vessels. Edema is a symptom of serious disease until proven otherwise, requiring complete medical evaluation and healthcare provider monitoring.

*Any undiagnosed edema requires medical evaluation.*

### WHAT CAUSES EDEMA?

Edema can occur as a result of certain situations (e.g., being pregnant, prolonged standing, or long airplane rides), obesity, age, or injury. Other conditions can cause swelling in one or both legs (e.g., "failure" of the heart, kidney, or liver; a blood clot in the leg; insulin resistance syndrome [IRS]; varicose veins; burns; bites; malnutrition; surgery).

*Certain medications may also cause your legs to swell. These include hormones (especially estrogen and testosterone), blood-pressure-lowering drugs, arthritis medication (including cortisone), diabetes medication, steroids, and antidepressants (e.g., MAOIs).*

### WHAT ROLE MIGHT CYTOKINES PLAY?

Fat tissue produces a cytokine protein (angiotensinogen) that causes salt retention. Synthesis or release of this protein can be induced by a single meal if high in calories, fat, and/or carbohydrates. Fluid retention is maintained chronically by continuing to eat a high-fat, high-sugar, high-calorie diet. Inflammatory cytokines damage small blood vessels and cause them to "leak" with resultant fluid retention. Cytokines also affect hormones secreted from the adrenal gland, heart, and brain that further promote fluid retention.

### WHAT RESULTS COULD I EXPECT FROM MNT?

Edema from any cause typically responds to the MNT Plan, usually by Food Phases 1 or 2. Patients taking diuretics (fluid pills) or vasodilators

## PRESCRIPTFIT
MEDICAL NUTRITION THERAPY ■ ■ ■ ■ ■ ■ ■

*Close medical supervision is required for those taking fluid, high blood pressure, or heart medication (see hypertension and congestive heart failure discussions beginning on pages 158 and 185, respectively).*

(heart or high blood pressure medication) should be very alert to hypotension (low blood pressure) in Food Phase 1 or 2. Rapid fluid loss may occur, requiring discontinuance of medication. After your edema subsides in Food Phase 1 and 2, stay alert for signs of relapse. Depending on cause, relapse may occur after a single meal of a higher fat, higher carbohydrate food or for other reasons (e.g., large salt intake, menstrual swelling, or certain arthritis medicine). Swelling should quickly resolve with resumption of Plan.

### How Can I Measure Symptom Change on the Plan?

*If you are taking prescription medicines, talk to your healthcare provider about when and how to cut down on what you take BEFORE you make any changes.*

Talk with your healthcare provider about what may be causing your swelling — cardiac illness, hypothyroidism, hypertension, OR perhaps a medication. If the latter, MNT will not reduce your symptoms; however, it can help determine if your edema is related to medication, depending on how quickly you see results without reducing medication dose or discontinuing altogether. Take a "baseline" measurement before beginning the Plan and again after each Food Phase or every four weeks.

**WHAT DO I NEED TO DO?**

1. *Grade the level of swelling you have on a scale from 0–10 (with "0" being no swelling at all to a "10" being severe edema).*

2. *Be sure to check the symptoms and grade your swelling AGAIN at the end of each Food Phase or every four weeks.*

3. *Take the results with you to your next medical appointment. Talk about how you're feeling and whether or not medications or other factors may be related to your swelling.*

**EDEMA DISEASE/SYMPTOM QUESTIONNAIRE**

| Level of Swelling | None                          Severe |
|---|---|
|  | 0  1  2  3  4  5  6  7  8  9  10 |

\* WARNING: Keep in close contact with your healthcare provider during initial phases of MNT; fluid loss could require immediate medication change to avoid hypotension.

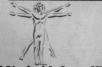

**PRESCRIPTFIT**
MEDICAL NUTRITION THERAPY ▪ ▪ ▪ ▪ ▪ ▪ ▪

# CHAPTER 10: ENHANCING WELLNESS

## FATIGUE

### WHAT IS FATIGUE?

Fatigue, characterized as physical and/or mental weariness, occurs either as a symptom of illness or as a side effect of medication. Normal fatigue occurs as a result of exertion, stress, or dealing with illness (e.g., "fighting off a cold").

### WHAT CAUSES FATIGUE?

Common, reversible causes of fatigue are sleep disorders, depression, cardiac disease of any cause, anemia, and hypothyroidism. Fatigue-related medication side effects include those from high blood pressure or depression medications as well as from antihistamines, sleeping medications, and anti-anxiety medications.

### WHAT ROLE MIGHT CYTOKINE IMBALANCE PLAY?

Cytokines most likely impact fatigue via disturbances in brain function with resultant sleep disturbances, such as sleep apnea. Additional fatigue occurs when there is a malfunction in the cardiopulmonary system that results in restless sleep due to poor breathing. Finally, fatigue may be due to "stress" hormones (adrenalin and cortisone) induced by excess cytokine production in fat and liver cells. Improvement in symptoms is clearly related to improvement in "toxic" cytokine levels (TNF, IL-1 and IL-6, CRP, and others).

### WHAT RESULTS COULD I EXPECT WITH MNT?

Fatigue often responds to the MNT Plan, regardless of cause. It is also one of the symptoms to return quickly with overeating/weight gain.

Fatigue is an important symptom to follow with each progressive Phase, typically responding to the first two Food Phases of the Plan.

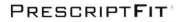

## PRESCRIPTFIT

MEDICAL NUTRITION THERAPY ■ ■ ■ ■ ■ ■ ■

# SECTION C: GETTING WELL...

As higher-calorie, higher-fat, and higher-carbohydrate Food Phases are added, a particular food group may be identified that produces increased fatigue, signalling that a food group should be avoided.

If you are experiencing fatigue as a result of medications, MNT will not reduce your symptoms. However, MNT can help you and your healthcare provider determine whether or not your fatigue is related to medication — if you don't see results within the first few weeks, and you are taking medication known for possible fatigue side effects, the chances are good that the medication is the culprit.

## HOW CAN I MEASURE SYMPTOM CHANGE ON THE PLAN?

First, you need to be clear about what may be causing your fatigue. Your healthcare provider may need to evaluate you for cardiac illness, hypothyroidism, anemia, or major depressive disorder.

Because many medications associated with fatigue side effects are prescribed for other conditions that respond to MNT, you and your healthcare provider may find (over time) that your need for these medications will diminish. Take a baseline measurement of your fatigue and re-measure after each Food Phase or every four weeks.

Most importantly, you (and your provider) need a way to measure progress over time. Talk with your healthcare provider at each regular visit about your symptoms and how they might change using the Plan. If you are taking prescription medicines, talk to your healthcare provider about when and how to cut down on what you take BEFORE you make any changes.

---

### WHAT DO I NEED TO DO?

1. Grade the level of energy you have on a scale from 0–10 (with "0" being no energy at all to a "10" being high energy).

2. Be sure to check the symptoms and grade your fatigue AGAIN at the end of each Food Phase or every four weeks.

3. Take the results with you to your next medical appointment. Talk about how you're feeling and whether or not medications may be related to your fatigue.

### FATIGUE DISEASE/SYMPTOM QUESTIONNAIRE

| Level of Fatigue | No energy         High energy<br>0  1  2  3  4  5  6  7  8  9  10 |
| --- | --- |

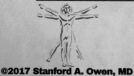

**PRESCRIPTFIT**
MEDICAL NUTRITION THERAPY ■ ■ ■ ■ ■ ■ ■

# ⇐ CHAPTER 10: ENHANCING WELLNESS ⇒

## FIBROMYALGIA

### WHAT IS FIBROMYALGIA?

Fibromyalgia is a complex chronic condition of unknown origin that affects women far more than men (80-90 percent), and those typically over 20 years of age. The condition involves pain in the muscles and soft tissue for which no diagnostic test can determine cause (e.g., blood tests, x-rays, MRI, CAT scan, etc.). Muscle and bone surfaces are typically most tender. Although fibromyalgia does not appear to shorten one's lifespan nor necessarily be physically debilitating, it is highly recurrent — full recovery is rare. However, with good support and treatment (usually involving some medication, good sleep habits, and exercise), fibromyalgia will not severely damage quality of life.

*Those with fibromyalgia tend to suffer from sleep disorders, depression, and anxiety.*

### WHAT CAUSES FIBROMYALGIA?

We really know very little about fibromyalgia; however, many theories exist regarding its cause. Some believe that the disorder is linked to viral infection, psychological disturbances or trauma, altered pain perception, lack of growth hormone, or lack of exercise. Other researchers point to change in sleep patterns or low levels of serotonin — a hormone that regulates moods and sleep. Research has shown that people with fibromyalgia tend to have disturbances in their deep sleep and different serotonin levels than others.

Female hormones are known to affect many brain and nerve neurotransmitters, including pain-mediating ones.

*Because of the prevalence of fibromyalgia among women (90 percent of those diagnosed), experts believe that the disorder is related in some way to female hormones.*

PRESCRIPT FIT®
MEDICAL NUTRITION THERAPY ▪ ▪ ▪ ▪ ▪ ▪ ▪

# ⌒ SECTION C: GETTING WELL... ⌒

### WHAT ROLE MIGHT CYTOKINE IMBALANCE PLAY?

Scientists point to Substance P (also known as neurokephlin) as a chemical in our bodies that modifies pain sensation in nerve fibers and brain cells.Because cytokines produced by fat cells influence production and function of Substance P, and female hormones regulate fat cell physiology, this link between obesity, cytokines, hormones, and pain regulation is very plausible.

### WHAT RESULTS COULD I EXPECT WITH MNT?

Cases of fibromyalgia improve, and even resolve, using the PrescriptFit MNT Plan, although response is difficult to predict. Most cases improve by Phase 1 or 2, especially when using the 7- or 14-day Food Phase Plan. You should see a change in symptoms by the end of week 4 if you rigidly adhere to the Plan.

Most patients experience improved sleep (and less fatigue) the quickest, followed by improved mood. Pain usually improves after sleep improves.

### HOW CAN I MEASURE SYMPTOM CHANGE ON THE PLAN?

Learn what may be causing your muscle pain and other symptoms. Visit your healthcare provider to determine whether or not you might have fibromyalgia. Talk with your healthcare provider about MNT and its impact on sleep, fatigue, depression, and other symptoms you're experiencing. Next, you want to have measurement of how severe each symptom is for you. This will give you a "baseline" to compare with future measurements.

Most importantly, you (and your provider) need a way to measure progress over time. Talk with your healthcare provider at each regular visit about your

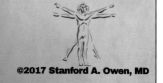

**PRESCRIPTFIT**®
MEDICAL NUTRITION THERAPY ▪ ▪ ▪ ▪ ▪ ▪ ▪

# ↦ CHAPTER 10: ENHANCING WELLNESS ↤

symptoms and how they might change using the Plan.

As with any medical condition, treatment traditionally means taking medications to reduce symptoms. You may find that as your symptoms lessen with MNT, you will need to take less medication OR perhaps discontinue pain medications entirely.

*If you are taking prescription medicines, ask your healthcare provider about when and how to cut down on what you take BEFORE you make any changes.*

## WHAT DO I NEED TO DO?

1.  *Check each symptom you are currently experiencing in the Disease/ Symptom Questionnaire below.*

2.  *Grade the level of pain you have on a scale from 0–10 (with "0" being no symptom at all to a "10" being severe and constant discomfort) as well as how often you need medication for the pain.*

3.  *Next, rate how you sleep (with "0" being "never sleep well" to "10," which indicates that you "always sleep well."*

4.  *Be sure to check the symptoms and grade your level of discomfort/sleep satisfaction AGAIN at the end of each Food Phase or every four weeks.*

5.  *Take the results with you to your next medical appointment. Talk about how you're feeling and whether or not you still need any prescription medications for fibromyalgia.*

6.  *Note if symptoms relapse with subsequent Food Phases or with off-Plan eating.*

### FIBROMYALGIA DISEASE/SYMPTOM QUESTIONNAIRE

| Symptom Experience | Level of Discomfort | | |
|---|---|---|---|
| **Pain** | **None** | | **Severe/Constant** |
|  | 0  1  2  3  4  5  6  7  8  9  10 | | |
| **Sleep** | **Never Well** | | **Always Well** |
|  | 0  1  2  3  4  5  6  7  8  9  10 | | |

\* WARNING: Never discontinue a prescribed medication without consulting with your healthcare provider.

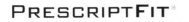

**PRESCRIPTFIT** ®
MEDICAL NUTRITION THERAPY ▪ ▪ ▪ ▪ ▪ ▪

# ⌐ SECTION C: GETTING WELL... ⌐

## INFERTILITY

### WHAT IS INFERTILITY?

Infertility is a complex disorder that occurs in both men and women. It is a disease of the reproductive system that prevents conception and can occur because of problems with any facet of the reproductive process.

### WHAT CAUSES INFERTILITY?

For women, most infertility cases stem from some problem with ovulation. Each step of the process from egg maturation to implantation may be influenced by dietary factors. There is an apparent relationship between infertility and obesity, especially in those who have insulin resistance syndrome (IRS).

*See pages 162 through 166 for discussion and disease/symptom tracking information for IRS.*

### WHAT ROLE MIGHT CYTOKINE IMBALANCE PLAY?

In the early 1990s, researchers discovered a hormone produced by fat cells, leptin, that helps regulate food intake and metabolism as well as fat storage in the cells. Subsequently, leptin was found to play a role in fertility. As excess nutrition and obesity develop, especially in insulin-resistant individuals, "resistance" to the action of leptin also develops.

*Although the link between cytokines and leptin has not been definitely established, the combination of weight loss and cytokine balance appears to be critical to positively influencing conception.*

### WHAT RESULTS COULD I EXPECT FROM MNT?

Although the link between MNT and fertility is not clear-cut, there appears to be one: Women with IRS (insulin resistant syndrome) are especially likely to benefit from MNT, partially because polycystic ovary syndrome is characterized, possibly even caused, by insulin resistance. Additionally, obesity influences leptin, a hormone important in regulating the entire process of conception.

*In addition to other possible hormonal and cytokine influences, leptin influences brain hormones involved in development, fertilization, and implantation of the egg as well as growth of the placenta.*

©2017 Stanford A. Owen, MD

# PRESCRIPTFIT
MEDICAL NUTRITION THERAPY ■ ■ ■ ■ ■ ■ ■

# ☞ CHAPTER 10: ENHANCING WELLNESS ☜

Many obese woman seen in our clinic for infertility who have been treated with MNT have conceived within three months, indicating that "the diet" and not "the obesity" contributed to the infertility. Women who are amennorrheic (without periods) may resume menstrual periods within the first eight weeks with rigid adherence to Food Phases 1 and 2 of the Plan.

*With MNT, those who are overweight as well as those who have IRS, polycystic ovary syndrome, or diabetes are the most likely to see results.*

## HOW CAN I MEASURE SYMPTOM CHANGE ON THE PLAN?

First of all, infertile couples should undergo evaluation by a fertility specialist prior to considering the PrescriptFit MNT Plan to determine possible causes and treatment solutions. Talk to the specialist about trying MNT prior to medication or other therapies.

Fertilization can best occur two weeks following a menstrual period when the woman ovulates. To better pinpoint when ovulation occurs, women can use:

*Unlike other illnesses discussed in this section, there is no Disease/Symptom Questionnaire for infertility. The important measurement is to pinpoint ovulation in one of the ways discussed at left.*

1. **Calendar tracking** — Record past menstrual cycle start date and duration to determine when you are most likely to be fertile.

*If appropriate, use the 14-day/phase Plan for best chances of fertility.*

2. **Taking basal body temperature** — Use a basal thermometer to check your body temperature each morning before becoming active. A rise of 0.4 to 1 degree Fahrenheit occurs when you ovulate.

3. **Checking vaginal mucus** — Daily test vaginal mucus for color (yellow, white, clear or cloudy), consistency (thick, sticky, or stretchy), and feel (dry, wet, sticky, slippery, stretchy). Ovulation probably occurs the same day that your mucus is clearest, most slippery, and most stretchy.

*Regular ovulation will not ensure conception. It is, however, a vital starting point. Work with your fertility specialist to optimize all the factors necessary to become pregnant.*

# PRESCRIPTFIT ®
MEDICAL NUTRITION THERAPY ▪ ▪ ▪ ▪ ▪ ▪ ▪

©2017 Stanford A. Owen, MD

# ⮞ Section C: Getting Well... ⮜

## Insomnia

### What is Insomnia?

People who suffer from insomnia get either too little sleep or the sleep they get is not very restful and refreshing. The problem doesn't necessarily have anything to do with the number of hours you sleep at night; it has to do with the quality of that sleep. For some, the problem is having trouble falling asleep in the first place. For others, the chronic tiredness comes from waking up too early in the morning. Some people fall asleep with no trouble, but wake up several times during the night and struggle to get back to sleep.

No matter what the pattern, insomnia leaves you feeling tired, sometimes even after "sleeping" seven to eight hours. This lack of adequate rest causes problems during the day: excessive sleepiness, fatigue, trouble thinking clearly or staying focused, or feeling depressed/irritable.

### What Causes Insomnia?

Insomnia may be a temporary problem induced by situational stress at home or at work, having a poor sleep environment (too much light, noise, or a partner who snores), or even certain medications. This type of short-term or occasional insomnia can last from a single night to a few weeks or occur from time to time.

If insomnia persists for at least three nights a week for over a month or more, you should see your healthcare provider about possible underlying medical causes. If this is not the case, your healthcare provider can help you identify patterns (working erratic shifts, not exercising, drinking caffeine or alcohol too close to bedtime, etc.) that might help positively alter your sleep patterns.

## PRESCRIPTFIT®
MEDICAL NUTRITION THERAPY ▪ ▪ ▪ ▪ ▪ ▪ ▪

# ~ CHAPTER 10: ENHANCING WELLNESS ~

## WHAT ROLE MIGHT CYTOKINE IMBALANCE PLAY?

How MNT improves insomnia is unknown. A majority of patients presenting to our clinic complain of insomnia. A majority improve sleep when following the Plan. Some improvement may be due to other related medical conditions, such as sleep apnea, acid reflux, or even improved oxygen exchange from better blood flow. No specific cytokines have been related to general insomnia related to anxiety. Perhaps, improved metabolism related to balanced cytokine production (see other disease sections) lowers adrenalin and cortisone levels, which are known to aggravate insomnia.

## WHAT RESULTS COULD I EXPECT WITH MNT?

Those suffering from insomnia often note improvement on the MNT Plan. Why this occurs is unknown; however, we suspect that improved brain function is related to improved nutrition or improved metabolism. Also, we know that branched-chain amino acids benefit patients suffering from a number of conditions that cause insomnia (depression, acid reflux, sleep apnea, arthritis, etc.), and not getting enough restful sleep complicates these conditions. Because of this interplay, you don't know if your insomnia got better because your arthritis symptoms eased (for example), or whether your arthritis symptoms improved because you're finally getting a good night's rest on a regular basis.

## HOW CAN I MEASURE SYMPTOM CHANGE ON THE PLAN?

First, you need to be clear about what might be causing your insomnia. Talk to your healthcare provider about your medical and sleep history. Find out if there's an underlying medical problem that needs attention.

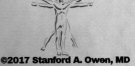

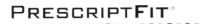

PRESCRIPTFIT®

MEDICAL NUTRITION THERAPY ▪ ▪ ▪ ▪ ▪ ▪ ▪

# SECTION C: GETTING WELL...

As with any medical condition, treatment may involve taking medications to reduce symptoms. You may find that as your symptoms lessen, you will need to take less medication OR perhaps discontinue your medications entirely. If you are taking prescription medicines, talk to your healthcare provider about when and how to cut down on what you take BEFORE you make any changes.

If you have chronic insomnia, you will want to measure how severe each symptom is for you. This will give you a "baseline" to compare with future measurements. Most importantly, you (and your provider) need a way to measure progress over time. Measure your symptoms again after four weeks or following each food phase. Take the results to your healthcare provider and discuss how your symptoms have changed using the Plan.

## WHAT DO I NEED TO DO?

1. Rate each symptom you are currently experiencing in the Disease/ Symptom Questionnaire below, noting how long it takes to fall asleep initially as well as how long you sleep before waking and then struggle to get back to sleep.

2. Be sure to check the symptoms and rate your level of sleeplessness AGAIN at the end of each Food Phase or every four weeks.

3. Take the results with you to your next medical appointment. Talk about how you're feeling and whether or not you still need any medications or other lifestyle changes to reduce your insomnia.

### INSOMNIA DISEASE/SYMPTOM QUESTIONNAIRE

| Symptom Experience | Level of Discomfort | | | | | | | |
|---|---|---|---|---|---|---|---|---|
| Difficulty falling asleep | **Average Minutes to Fall Asleep** | | | | | | | |
| | 1 | 5 | 10 | 15 | 30 | 60 | 120 | 180 |
| Times awakened after initial sleep established | **Number of Instances** | | | | | | | |
| | 1 | 2 | 3 | 4 | 5 | 6 | 7 | 8 |
| Length of time to reestablish sleep | **Average Minutes** | | | | | | | |
| | 1 | 5 | 10 | 15 | 30 | 60 | 120 | 180 |

# PRESCRIPTFIT
MEDICAL NUTRITION THERAPY ▪ ▪ ▪ ▪ ▪ ▪ ▪

# ☞ CHAPTER 10: ENHANCING WELLNESS ☜

## JOINT PAIN (HIP, KNEE, FEET)

### WHAT IS JOINT PAIN?

Joint pain in the hip, knee, or feet all typically occur in those who are obese. The joints associated with these areas bear the weight of our frame and help to keep us upright. Stress on these joints as our bodies adapt to changes in weight and body shape can lead to often-debilitating discomfort.

The most common joint complaint is **knee pain.** The knee bears the brunt of increased weight and abnormal angle-stress from obesity. The knee is also subject to sudden twists and bends of unexpected slips and falls.Minor tears in the ligaments, tendons, and cartilage (that result from these slips and falls) promote inflammation and swelling.

**Foot pain** is a frequent complaint of obese patients. Foot pain can arise from the ankle joint, the nerves to the foot, and ligaments (plantar fasciitis or heel spur). All three conditions are more common in obesity for the same reasons noted with knee pain. The human foot was designed to bear weight down the shank of the leg and heel, rather than towards the toes (as it must do in obesity because of having a larger abdomen).

*Be sure to see a healthcare provider familiar with foot pain for accurate diagnosis.*

**Hip pain** is the least frequent and most severe type of joint damage related to obesity. Pain from the hip joint is typically felt on the front of the hip. Hip pain requires expert diagnosis and rehab; you will need to see a joint specialist and possibly a physical therapist as well.

### WHAT CAUSES JOINT PAIN?

Joint pain and obesity are bedfellows. Joint pain

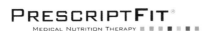

PRESCRIPTFIT®
MEDICAL NUTRITION THERAPY ∎ ∎ ∎ ∎ ∎ ∎ ∎

©2017 Stanford A. Owen, MD

# ≈ Section C: Getting Well... ≈

may occur from increased strain and tearing of joint support (ligament, tendon, cartilage, bone) due to excessive weight and from abnormal joint angles from distorted weight distribution.

On another level, joint pain is related to your body's ability to repair damaged collagen — the support protein for the ligaments, tendons, cartilage, and bone. Obesity is associated with changes in your body's hormone levels — the ones that impact your ability to repair collagen. Those who are obese tend to have low testosterone levels and low growth hormone levels, both of which are essential to collagen repair. Obesity is also associated with elevated levels of cortisone, which destroys collagen. As we age, our ability to repair damaged collagen also decreases, making obesity and aging a very troubling combination.

## What Role Might Cytokine Imbalance Play?

Fat cells produce cytokines that promote immune inflammation that damages joint structures. The combination of increased weight, abnormal angles of movement, and increased immune damage with diminished collagen repair destroys joints and causes pain with disability. Those who are obese have more problems with joint injury because their bodies produce too much of a protein enzyme (metalloproteases) that destroys collagen. Since overproduction of this enzyme is linked to out-of-balance cytokines, PrescriptFit can offer significant benefits.

## What Results Could I Expect with MNT?

**Knee pain** often improves with the MNT Plan via decreased weight and diminished inflammation.

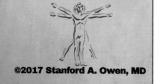

PRESCRIPTFIT®
MEDICAL NUTRITION THERAPY ▪ ▪ ▪ ▪ ▪ ▪ ▪

# CHAPTER 10: ENHANCING WELLNESS

In our clinic, decreased pain and medication requirements are seen long before major weight changes. Expert rehabilitation is vital. Abdominal weakness is just as important as obesity in promoting abnormal knee-angle stress. "Ab" strengthening should be a practiced daily in those with back, hip, knee, or foot pain.

For improving **foot pain**, the Plan fosters weight loss and positive changes to posture that occur with reducing abdomen size. In addition, exercise and physical therapy as well as heel pads and arch supports will likely speed recovery. In our clinic, those using the MNT Plan often note improvement in foot pain, although usually at a slower rate than those experiencing improvement in knee pain.

*Those with hip pain are probably less likely to improve using the Plan. However, diminished weight and decreased abdominal protuberance helps all joints below the pelvis.*

## How Can I Measure Symptom Change on the Plan?

First, you need to be clear about what might be causing your joint pain. Talk to your healthcare provider about the type of pain you have, when you first noticed it, the severity, and what treatment combination might be best for you. Next, you want to have a measurement of how severe the joint pain is for you. This will give you a "baseline" to compare with future measurements.

Most importantly, you (and your provider) need a way to measure progress over time. Talk with your healthcare provider at each regular visit about your symptoms and how they might change using the Plan.

As with any medical condition, treatment traditionally means taking medications to reduce symptoms. A number of prescription and over-the-counter pain medications can be taken to reduce symptoms. You may find that as your symptoms lessen, you will need to take less medication OR

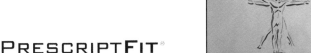

**PRESCRIPTFIT**®
MEDICAL NUTRITION THERAPY ▪ ▪ ▪ ▪ ▪ ▪ ▪

## ⌒ SECTION C: GETTING WELL... ⌒

perhaps discontinue your medications entirely. If you are taking prescription medicines, talk to your healthcare provider about when and how to cut down on what you take BEFORE you make any changes.

### WHAT DO I NEED TO DO?

1. Using the Disease/Symptom Questionnaire below, indicate for each type of joint pain you have (knee, foot, hip) the severity initially on a scale from 0–10 (with "0" being no symptom at all to a "10" being severe discomfort).

2. Be sure to check the symptoms and grade your level of discomfort AGAIN at the end of each 12 weeks.

3. Record the number of medications you currently take for each type of joint pain initially when beginning MNT and again after 12 weeks.

4. Take the results with you to your next medical appointment. Talk about how you're feeling and whether or not you still need to take medications for joint pain.

#### JOINT PAIN DISEASE/SYMPTOM QUESTIONNAIRE

| Initial Knee Pain | Knee Pain at 12 Weeks |
|---|---|
| Mild      Severe | Mild      Severe |
| 1 2 3 4 5 6 7 8 9 10 | 1 2 3 4 5 6 7 8 9 10 |
| Initial Foot Pain | Foot Pain at 12 Weeks |
| Mild      Severe | Mild      Severe |
| 1 2 3 4 5 6 7 8 9 10 | 1 2 3 4 5 6 7 8 9 10 |
| Initial Hip Pain | Hip Pain at 12 Weeks |
| Mild      Severe | Mild      Severe |
| 1 2 3 4 5 6 7 8 9 10 | 1 2 3 4 5 6 7 8 9 10 |

**Number of Medications Used** \_\_\_\_
**(e.g., Tylenol™ + Ibuprofen = 2)**

\* WARNING: Never discontinue a prescribed medication without consulting with your healthcare provider.

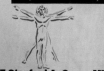

©2017 Stanford A. Owen, MD

**PRESCRIPTFIT**
MEDICAL NUTRITION THERAPY ▪ ▪ ▪ ▪ ▪ ▪ ▪

## MIKE & BOB —
## WEIGHT LOSS IS IRRELEVANT!

Read the stories below and on the next page about Mike and Bob, two patients for whom nutrition therapy, not weight loss, was the key to getting well.

**Mike was referred to us by his doctor for treatment of severe type 2 diabetes. His blood sugar was consistently over 300, and he had lost 80 pounds over the previous year.** Mike was now 6'1" and weighed 160 pounds, looking much like a concentration camp survivor. His nerve fibers were dead and dying with numbness from his toes to his knees, and his intestinal nerves were dying, which caused uncontrollable vomiting after eating — just another factor in his inability to gain weight. Because his muscles cramped constantly, and he could barely walk, Mike had had to give up his job as a boat mechanic.

Mike was already on the highest doses he could take of several oral medications with insulin his only remaining option. His doctor knew of PrescriptFit and wanted to see if I could help. With detailed cautions, I explained that we could try Medical Nutrition Therapy and that I would follow his case closely.

Because Mike was malnourished, I started him on 1200 calories/day of PrescriptFit shakes and soup products and all the food he could tolerate in Food Phases 2-7 (seafood, poultry, vegetables, eggs, nuts, and whole fruit). He felt much better in just three days and gained six pounds his first week. His blood sugar decreased by the end of the first week and normalized after six weeks. Mike remained on his metformin and Avandia™ (since taken off the market) and eventually gained 50 pounds. His neuropathy (both gut nerves and extremities) completely reversed. Mike was able to return to his job after his muscle cramps went away (in just seven days) and his strength returned.

For over seven years, Mike has avoided taking insulin and lived a "normal" life. His only treatment difference? Medical Nutrition Therapy with PrescriptFit. His biggest challenge has been discovering how to enjoy his "Splurge" meal limits without adversely affecting his blood sugar.

**When Bob first came to my clinic in March of 2004, he was 64 and had been suffering with congestive heart failure (CHF) for three years.** He had been in the hospital five times in that three years and had had a heart stent three months prior to my evaluation.

*Continued on page 212...*

# PRESCRIPTFIT®
MEDICAL NUTRITION THERAPY ▪ ▪ ▪ ▪ ▪ ▪ ▪

©2017 Stanford A. Owen, MD

# ~ SECTION C: GETTING WELL... ~

...Continued from page 211

Bob was critically ill! His diabetes A1C was 8.6. His kidneys were failing (BUN 85, creatinine 3.8), and his feet were massively swollen, red, and thickened, with skin ulcers and fluid oozing into his socks. He had seen a vascular surgeon for placement of a kidney dialysis shunt and actually came to me because he wanted to improve prior to having shunt surgery.

I placed Bob on PrescriptFit shakes ONLY for three months at a level of 800-1000 calories/day. He immediately lost 20 pounds of fluid, and his legs quit weeping fluid. His breathlessness also improved immediately, and he began a slow walking program. After 12 weeks, Bob had lost 40 pounds, and his heart failure improved (ejection fraction increased from 32 to 56 percent). Most impressively, Bob's kidney function improved (BUN reduced from 85 to 36 and creatinine from 3.8 to 1.7), making it possible for him to avoid having to go on dialysis. His blood sugar normalized to an A1C of 5.6.

We added in one food group at a time every two weeks while closely monitoring heart and kidney function. Working with his physician, Bob discontinued five of his nine medications including Lasix (fluid pills), hypertension medication (except captopril), and all of his diabetes medication.

What's happened to Bob since then? After making a large amount of money on a stock tip, he traveled to Europe and walked in the Alps without difficulty. He witnessed the birth and growth of his grandchildren. As of October 2013 (at age 73), he had never re-entered the hospital, never had dialysis (kidneys are now at BUN 25 and creatinine 1.4). His only treatment? Medical Nutrition Therapy with PrescriptFit.

Bob is a prime example of how it's not the weight, its' the diet! His weight is 236 (down from 260), but he's still 76 pounds heavier than his military weight of 160. Bob is still obese but diligently follows PrescriptFit diet strategy.

While I can present countless, similar cases, these results may not be reproducible in all cases, have not been verified by the Food and Drug Administration, and may not be reproducible with those practitioners who have less experience with MNT. What these cases DO reveal is that MNT should be considered in cases like these (those with diabetes and hypertension especially) where professional guidelines clearly support MNT as first and primary treatment. Oh so often, MNT is completely ignored or offered only halfheartedly. We hope to bring all patients appropriate care through their personal physicians using Medical Nutrition Therapy, including PrescriptFit.

**CASE STUDIES**

**PRESCRIPTFIT**®
MEDICAL NUTRITION THERAPY ▪ ▪ ▪ ▪ ▪ ▪ ▪

# NOTES

QUESTIONS?

EMAIL DR. OWEN AT
DROWENMD@DRDIET.COM

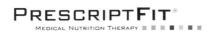

# NOTES

**QUESTIONS?**

EMAIL DR. OWEN AT
DROWENMD@DRDIET.COM

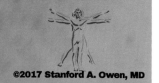

**PRESCRIPTFIT** ®

MEDICAL NUTRITION THERAPY

# APPENDIX A:
# FAT TISSUE & CYTOKINES

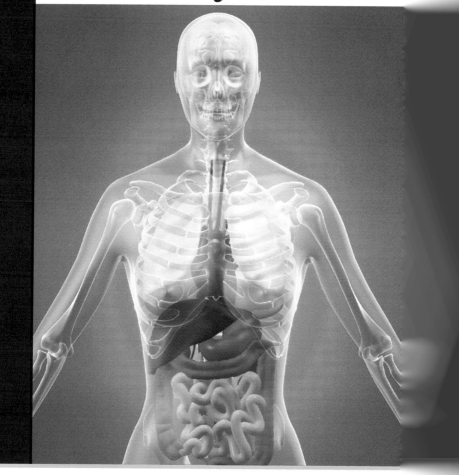

Why PrescriptFit® works to reduce disease symptoms and promote weight loss lies in the relationship between fat cells, cytokines, and branched chain amino acids. Below are some definitions to help you understand these relationships. Be sure to talk to your healthcare provider about cytokines and the impact of fat cells on your overall health.

## ADIPOKINE

See pages 218 through 219 for a list of common adipokines and their functions.

A cytokine produced by adipose (fat) cells. A short list of known adipokines includes adiponectin, resistin, leptin, tumor necrosis factor, angiotensinogen, interleukin 1,2,6,18, plasminogen activator inhibitor–1 (PAI–1), macrophage inhibiting factor, adipsin, free fatty acids, and growth factors.

## BRANCHED CHAIN AMINO ACIDS

Leucine, isoleucine, and valine are the primary branched chain amino acids. They are called "branched" due to their chemical structure. These amino acids, plus threonine and lysine, comprise 75 percent of amino acids used for energy metabolism or protein synthesis. The ratio of each amino acid affects the metabolism of other amino acids. Therefore, achieving balance of the key amino acids can improve energy and protein metabolism.

## CYTOKINES

Protein molecules (peptides) made by cells of the immune system, fat cells, and other organs that regulate inflammation, metabolism, cell growth, vascular tone, blood cell formation, and behavior. Cytokines made by fat cells are called "adipokines" (from an adipose cell). Key characteristics of cytokines are that they:

> **Have multiple functions:** The same cytokine may regulate inflammation, blood vessel function, or infertility.

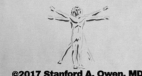

PRESCRIPTFIT®
MEDICAL NUTRITION THERAPY ▪ ▪ ▪ ▪ ▪ ▪ ▪

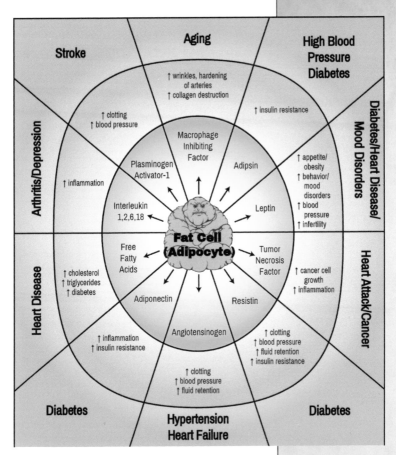

> **Are redundant:** Different cytokines may have the same function.

> **Work in a cascading manner:** One cytokine released may trigger the next, then another, and another, resulting in many different reactions in different organs.

> **May come from different organs:** Multiple organs make the same cytokines (e.g., leptin may be made by fat cells, brain tissue, or the intestine).

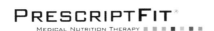

PRESCRIPTFIT
MEDICAL NUTRITION THERAPY

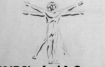

©2017 Stanford A. Owen, MD

# COMMON ADIPOKINES

### ADIPONECTIN

A prevalent and protective cytokine — Higher levels of adiponectin prevent heart disease and diabetes. Lower levels are produced by obesity, high fat, high sugar diets, inactivity, and inflammation from other diseases (arthritis).

### ADIPSIN

Made by abdominal fat cells, this cytokine promotes insulin resistance and fluid retention. It also activates other inflammatory cytokines.

### ANGIOTENSINOGEN

A cytokine that regulates blood pressure and fluid balance, inflammation of blood vessels, and growth of fat cells.

### GROWTH FACTORS

A host of cytokines that make cells grow (including cancer cells). Epidermal growth factor produces thickening of skin cells, especially on the neck and arm pits, causing darkening of the skin (acanthosis nigricans) and skin tags.

### FREE FATTY ACIDS (FFA)

Triglycerides released by fat cells that float to the liver or muscle and are used as energy. When excess FFA is formed, it causes insulin resistance, muscle malfunction, and cytokine formation.

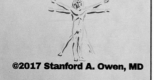

PRESCRIPTFIT®
MEDICAL NUTRITION THERAPY ▪ ▪ ▪ ▪ ▪ ▪ ▪

## INTERLEUKIN 1, 2, 6, AND 18

Cytokines that regulate inflammation and immune function. Levels rise with obesity, high fat, high sugar diets, and other diseases of inflammation.

## LEPTIN

The first discovered adipokine — Leptin regulates eating behavior, blood vessel function, immune function, fertility, and at least 30 other functions.

## MACROPHAGE INHIBITING FACTOR (MIF)

A cytokine that promotes macrophage (white blood cells that ingest foreign material) attack on arteries and into fat tissue.

## PLASMINOGEN ACTIVATOR INHIBITOR-1 (PAI-1)

Cytokine that promotes clotting and thrombosis. Increases in obesity, high fat, high sugar diets. PAI-1 levels can reduce by 50% in one week on VLCD (very low calorie diets).

## RESISTIN

Cytokine with opposite effects of adiponectin — Resistin causes "resistance" to the action of insulin in cell function.

## TUMOR NECROSIS FACTOR (TNF)

A cytokine that regulates inflammation and immune function, including cancer control. TNF has a role in energy balance, insulin resistance and diabetes, fat metabolism, and blood vessel damage. Obesity and high-fat, high-sugar diets increase levels and function of TNF. Elevated TNF lowers adiponectin levels.

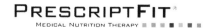

# NOTES

**QUESTIONS?**

EMAIL DR. OWEN AT
DROWENMD@DRDIET.COM

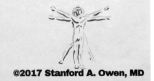

**PRESCRIPTFIT®**
MEDICAL NUTRITION THERAPY

# Appendix B: Calorie Math

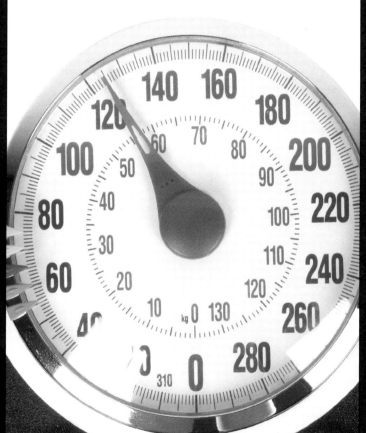

# CALORIE MATH

*Use the notes page at the end of this appendix to list those foods that you like (or are willing to experiment with) that "add up" to be the best "bang for your calorie buck."*

Review the chart below and on the following page to see how the foods you eat "add up" to extra exercise in order to burn those calories. For example, is having fried shrimp rather than shrimp cocktail worth an extra mile of walking for every ounce you eat? Do the math; it will be a real eye-opener!

| FOOD ITEM | CALORIES/ OUNCE | # OUNCES = 1 MILE OF WALKING* |
|---|---|---|
| Beef | 100–125 | .75–1 |
| Pork | 100–150 | .5–1 |
| Seafood (grilled, baked, etc.) | 25–30 | 4 |
| Seafood (fried) | 125 | .75 |
| Poultry (skinless, not fried) | 50 | 2 |
| Poultry (skin on) | 75–100 | 1–1.25 |
| Poultry (fried) | 100–125 | .75–1 |
| Eggs (EACH) | 1 Egg = 100 oz. | 1 Egg = 1 Mile |
| Nuts | 175 | .57 |
| **Fruits** | | |
| lemon, tomato | 5 | 20 |
| melon | 10 | 10 |
| apple, pineapple, orange | 15 | 9 |
| grapes | 20 | 5 |
| banana | 30 | 3 |
| avocado | 45 | 2 |
| dried fruit | 85 | 1–1.2 |
| **Starches** | | |
| chips | 125–150 | .5–.75 |
| bread | 80 | 1–1.2 |
| muffins/cereal | 100 | 1 |
| pastries/cake | 125 | .75 |
| pie | 150 | .5 |

**PRESCRIPTFIT**®
MEDICAL NUTRITION THERAPY ▪ ▪ ▪ ▪ ▪ ▪ ▪

| FOOD ITEM | CALORIES/ OUNCE | # OUNCES = 1 MILE OF WALKING* |
|---|---|---|
| **Beverages** | | |
| soft drinks (sweetened) | 12 | 8–9 |
| beer | 12 | 8–9 |
| wine | 20 | 5 |
| liquor (scotch, rum, etc.) | 60 | 1.67 |
| liqueur (brandy, kahlua, etc.) | 100–150 | .5–1 |
| juice/whole milk | 20 | 5 |
| **Dairy** | | |
| non-fat cottage cheese | 25 | 4 |
| yogurt | 25–50 | 2–4 |
| sour cream | 30–50 | 2–4 |
| cream cheese | 50–75 | 2–2.5 |
| cheese | 25–100 | 1–4 |
| ice cream | 125–150 | .5–.75 |
| milk | 20 | 5 |
| cream | 75 | 1.25 |

| FOOD ITEM | CALORIES/ CUP | # CUPS = 1 MILE OF WALKING* |
|---|---|---|
| **Vegetables** | | |
| leafy, green (bell pepper, celery, lettuce, summer squash) | 10–20 | 5–10 |
| onions, carrots, asparagus, okra, green beans, cauliflower, broccoli | 40–60 | 2–3 |
| winter squash, peas (fresh), stewed tomatoes, diced tomatoes | 80–120 | .8–1.25 |
| corn, mashed potatoes, rice, dried peas, beans | 140–200 | .5–.71 |

\* One mile of walking/day (15 minutes) burns approximately 100 calories in a 150-pound individual.

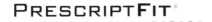

PRESCRIPTFIT®
MEDICAL NUTRITION THERAPY ■ ■ ■ ■ ■ ■ ■ ■

# NOTES

**QUESTIONS?**

**EMAIL DR. OWEN AT
DROWENMD@DRDIET.COM**

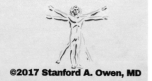

**PRESCRIPTFIT**®
MEDICAL NUTRITION THERAPY

# Appendix C:
# Food Addiction
# & Medication

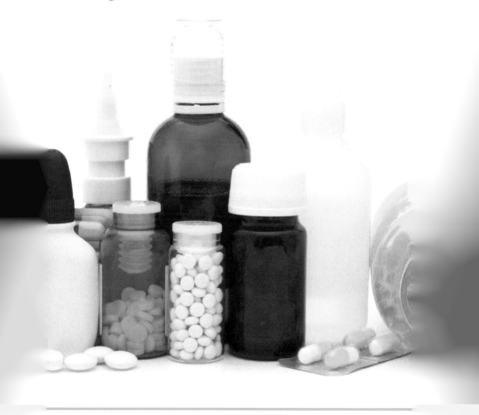

# NOTES:

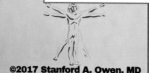

PRESCRIPT**FIT**®
MEDICAL NUTRITION THERAPY ▪ ▪ ▪ ▪ ▪ ▪ ▪

# MEDICATIONS THAT ALTER CASH (CRAVINGS, APPETITE, SATIETY, HUNGER)

| Class | Generic Name | Brand Name |
|---|---|---|
| Corticosteroids | • prednisone<br>• triamcinolone (cream)<br>• clobetasol (cream<br>• tiamcinolone (injection<br>• dexamethasone (injection)<br>• beclomethazone (inhaler) | • Multiple<br>• Multiple<br>• Multiple<br>• Celestone/Kenalog<br>• Decadron<br><br>• Advair, Arnuity Ellipta, Asmanex, Azmacort, Dulera, Flovent, Pulmicort, Symbicort, Qvar |
| Antidepressants | • paroxetine<br>• fluoxetine<br>• venlafaxine<br>• sertraline<br>• duloxitine<br>• mertazapine<br>• trazadone<br>• amitriptyline<br>• protriptyline<br>• nortriptyline | • Paxil, Paxil CR<br>• Prosac, Sarafem, Pexeva<br>• Effexor<br>• Zoloft<br>• Cymbalta<br>• Remeron, Remeron SolTab<br>• Desyrel, apo-Trazadone, Oleptro<br>• Elavil/Triavil, Endep, Levate<br>• Vivactil<br>• Pamelor |
| Antipsychotics | • olanzapine<br>• clozapine<br>• risperadone<br>• quetiapine<br>• ziprazidone<br>• aripiprezole<br>• holoperidol<br>• thiothixene<br>• asenapine | • Zyprexa<br>• Clonzanil<br>• Risperdol<br>• Seroquel<br>• Geodon<br>• Abilify<br>• Haldol<br>• Navane<br>• Safris |

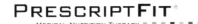

PRESCRIPTFIT®
MEDICAL NUTRITION THERAPY ▪ ▪ ▪ ▪ ▪ ▪ ▪

©2017 Stanford A. Owen, MD

| Class | Generic Name | Brand Name |
|---|---|---|
| Anti-epileptics | • valpriate<br>• carbamazine<br>• gabapentin<br>• vigabatrin<br>• levetiracetam<br>• oxycarbazepine<br>• tiagabine<br>• lamotrigene | • Depakote<br>• Tegretol<br>• Neruontin<br>• Lyrica<br>• Keppra<br>• Trileptal<br>• Gabitril<br>• Lamictal |
| Mood Stabilizers | • lithium<br>• anti-epileptics (see above) | |
| Pain Medication | • gabapentin<br>• levetiracetam<br>• opiates<br>  — codeine<br>  — fentanyl<br>  — hydrocodone<br>  — hydromorphone<br>  — meperidine<br>  — methadone<br>  — morphine<br><br>  — oxycodone<br><br>  — oxycodone and naloxone | • Neurontin<br>• Lyrica<br>• Multiple:<br>  — Only available in generic form<br>  — Actiq, Duragesic, Fentora<br>  — Lorcet, Lortab, Norco, Vicodin<br>  — Dilaudid, Exalgo<br>  — Demerol<br>  — Dolophine, Methadose<br>  — Avinza, Kadian, MS Contin, Ora-Morph SR<br>  — OxyContin, Oxyfast, Percocet, Roxicodone<br>  — Targiniq ER |
| Antihistamines | • Diphendydramine<br>• Certrizine<br>• Loratidine<br>• Fexofenadine<br>• Chlorpheniramine<br><br>• Doxepin<br>• Hydroxyzine | • Benedryl<br>• Zertec<br>• Claritin<br>• Allegra<br>• Chlor-trimeton, Allergy Relief, Chlorphen, Aller-Chlor<br>• Deptran, Sinequan<br>• Atarax |

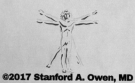

PRESCRIPT**FIT**®
MEDICAL NUTRITION THERAPY ▪ ▪ ▪ ▪ ▪ ▪ ▪

| Class | Generic Name | Brand Name |
|---|---|---|
| Diabetes Medications | • insulin<br>• sulfonylureas:<br>  — glibenclamide<br>  — glimepiride<br>  — glipizide<br>  — tolbutamide<br>  — chlorpropamide<br>  — tolazamide<br>  — glyburide/metformin<br>  — glipizide/Metformin<br>  — pioglitazone/ glimepiride<br>  — rosiglitazone/ glimepiride<br>• glitazone | • Multiple<br>• Multiple:<br>  — Micronase, DiaBeta, Glynase, PresTab<br>  — Amaryl<br>  — Glucotrol, Glucotrol XL<br><br><br>  — Tolinase<br>  — Glucovance<br>  — Metaglip<br>  — Duetact<br><br>  — Avandaryl<br><br>• Actos |
| Weight Loss/Appetite Control Medications | • Pheteramine/ topiramate*<br>• Locerserin*<br>• Bupropion/naltrexon*<br>• H2 blockers<br>• Metformin<br>• GLP-1 agonists*:<br>  — liraglutide<br>  — albigludtide<br>  — exenatide<br>  — lixisenatide | • Osymia*<br><br>• Belviq*<br>• Contrave*<br>• Cimetidine/Ranitidine/Famotidine<br>• Glucophage<br><br>  — Victoza*<br>  — Tanzeum<br>  — Bydureon<br>  — Lyxumia (EU approved) |

*FDA approved for weight loss

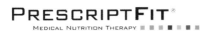

PRESCRIPTFIT®
MEDICAL NUTRITION THERAPY ■ ■ ■ ■ ■ ■ ■

# NOTES

**QUESTIONS?**

EMAIL DR. OWEN AT
DROWENMD@DRDIET.COM

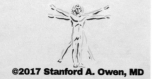
**PRESCRIPTFIT**®
MEDICAL NUTRITION THERAPY

# APPENDIX D:
# HEALTHCARE PROVIDER
# RESOURCES

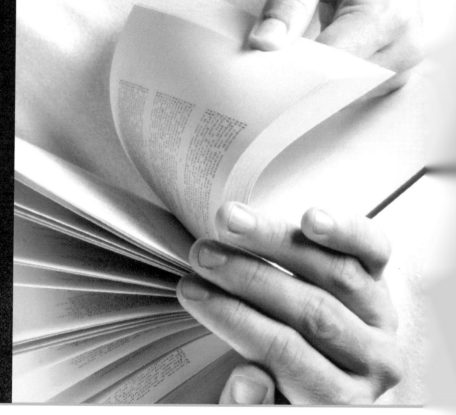

# HEALTHCARE PROVIDER FAQS

### HOW FAST DOES ONE SEE RESPONSES?

Responses vary depending on the medical condition and its severity, additional illnesses, and medications prescribed. The more severe the symptoms, the faster and more dramatic the response. Those individuals with few medical problems and a minimal amount of weight to lose will note the least dramatic "benefit." Most symptoms respond within several weeks.

### WHICH DISEASES RESPOND MOST PREDICTABLY?

Using over a decade of practice-based experience and measuring outcomes data, we've found diseases that usually respond quickly and dramatically are Type 2 diabetes, GERD (acid reflux), edema (swelling), fatigue, dyspnea (breathlessness), CHF (congestive heart failure), and irritable bowel syndrome. Slower and less-dramatic responses occur with steatosis (fatty liver), headache, joint and back pain, hypertension, hyperlipidemia, and sleep apnea. Least-predictable improvement occurs with asthma, angina, arthritis (inflammatory type), depression, fibromyalgia, and insomnia.

### WHAT ARE EXPECTED SIDE EFFECTS OF THE DIET, AND HOW ARE THEY MANAGED?

Most common side effects are gas and diarrhea, managed by using Lactose Free PrescriptFit® products. Weakness occurs when blood pressure or diabetes medications are not tapered or stopped fast enough. Most physicians are surprised by the degree and rate of improvement and often cite "the diet" rather than the necessary medication adjustments when side effects occur. Constipation is occasionally a problem, usually solved by adding fiber (Citrucel®), stool softeners, or Fish Oil (Omega III). Laxatives are usually unnecessary.

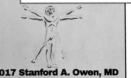

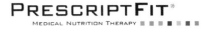

PRESCRIPTFIT®
MEDICAL NUTRITION THERAPY ■ ■ ■ ■ ■ ■ ■

## How does this diet compare to traditional national dietary guidelines? How does it differ and are those differences a problem?

PrescriptFit reflects traditional nutrition guidelines by promoting leaner foods for everyday consumption. The differences are sequentially adding food groups and lack of portion control. The sequential strategy can be safely used since the PrescriptFit products provide complete nutrition. Portion control is unnecessary since the PrescriptFit products taken prior to meals result in less total calorie consumption and improved metabolism of foods consumed. Another important difference is that the diet fosters learning about food group nutrition while experiencing how adding each food group impacts medical symptoms.

## When is close medical supervision recommended/required?

Whenever a medical condition exists that requires adjustment of medication, especially diabetes, congestive heart failure, hypertension, and edema (swelling). These conditions require close monitoring and medication adjustment. Other medical conditions usually need adjustment less urgently. Monitor all individuals following the 14-day/Phase Plan.

## How can a healthcare provider contact us with questions?

Contact us anytime via www.drdiet.com or by phone (888-460-6286) to speak with a qualified healthcare provider. A direct call will always be answered or returned.

## What published findings support this approach?

A number of journal articles have been published on specific impacts of amino acids and cytokine imbalance on specific diseases (e.g., metabolic syndrome, type 2 diabetes, cardiovascular disease, mental health disorders). These articles have been included in this

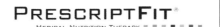

PRESCRIPTFIT®
MEDICAL NUTRITION THERAPY ■ ■ ■ ■ ■ ■ ■

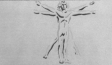

©2017 Stanford A. Owen, MD

appendix (see pages 237–239). Unfortunately, most of this research has not focused on disease versus specific diet approaches, and no diets have been researched with multiple diseases concurrently. Few have correlated specific changes in cytokines with specific diseases using a specific diet. Published research does not seem to reflect what Dr. Owen has done in the past decade — look at multiple diseases, measure specific cytokines (mostly CRP), and do so on a diet time line (most measure weight loss as the measure of benefit rather than symptom reduction).

PrescriptFit products were developed by a physician in private practice who is also a physician nutrition specialist (see "What is a Physician Nutrition Specialist" FAQ on the next page) without funding from major pharmaceutical companies or food manufacturers. The cost of performing scientific studies that would satisfy publication requirements for most peer-reviewed journals is astronomical. However, efforts are underway to secure grants for formal studies since the impact on health is, in our opinion, so substantial for such minimal cost and risk.

### WHAT PRACTICE-BASED FINDINGS PROMOTE PRESCRIPTFIT MEDICAL NUTRITION THERAPY?

In 1995, Dr. Owen started measuring multiple end points when patients followed the HMR very low calorie diet (VLCD). By 1997, he had a large enough experience base (>1,500 patients) to start a computer-based data system. By 2000, he had measures on all the disease parameters covered in section C of this book. As data emerged demonstrating benefit of branched-chain amino acids, the PrescriptFit products were developed to maximize and improve outcomes seen with the VLCD plans. Data since 2000 has been collected using the progressive PrescriptFit Food Phase plan with similar results.

### HOW WERE THE CLINICAL OUTCOME MEASURES DEVELOPED?

In the early 1990s, Dr. Owen's clinic developed a computerized data entry system to measure improvement in disease conditions

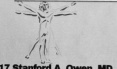

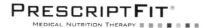

PRESCRIPTFIT®
MEDICAL NUTRITION THERAPY ▪ ▪ ▪ ▪ ▪ ▪ ▪

witnessed daily. The data allowed a more objective way to prove the benefit and to improve methods and products. After development of measures for the obvious disease targets, they realized that many less-obvious conditions and symptoms responded as well. The result of the data system is the Symptom Score Sheet used in the PrescriptFit Calendar.

## WHAT IS A PHYSICIAN NUTRITION SPECIALIST?

A Physician Nutrition Specialist is someone who has studied in the field of nutrition for a specified time, has contributed to the nutrition sciences on a professional level, has passed a Board Certification Exam, and then been accepted by that Board as a Certified Member. Dr. Stanford Owen was one of fewer than 100 physicians certified in the initial board applications of 2001, the first year of formal Board formation. He is accepted as a Fellow in the North American Association for the Study of Obesity — an honor requiring that one contribute significantly to the published, clinical, or socioeconomic issues relating to obesity and nutrition. Few Board Certified Physician Nutrition Specialists have developed commercially available nutrition therapy plans. None have measured outcome as a component of a medical nutrition therapy program — Dr. Owen's life-long mission.

## WHAT MEDICATION-BALANCING ISSUES ARE IMPORTANT FOR PATIENTS USING MNT?

For patients taking medication for diabetes, hypertension, or fluid retention, the need to down-regulate these medications occurs rapidly, and patients will get symptomatic (even dangerously symptomatic) if not monitored closely.

## WHAT ROLE DO THE INDIVIDUAL FOOD PHASES PLAY IN DIET SUCCESS AND SYMPTOM MEDIATION?

Sequentially adding each food group promotes education: learning how each food group specifically impacts medical symptoms and how to buy, cook, and flavor specific foods for a specific time period.

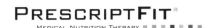

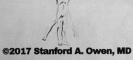

This education promotes long-term eating habit changes and validates the patient's experience about what makes them feel better and what doesn't.

Additionally, each food group has nutritional characteristics that predict benefit or harm to physiology (in terms of calories, percent protein, percent fat and type of fat, percent carbs and type of carbs) — all specific to individual physiology. For example, a patient who is diabetic with hypertension and high lipids might hate vegetables and seafood. His wife wants to be a vegetarian. This could pose a real dilemma for adding some of the food groups; however, the built-in flexibility of PrescriptFit MNT allows for skipping some of the early Food Phases or reordering them to accommodate these types of dilemmas.

### HOW OFTEN SHOULD FOLLOW-UP APPOINTMENTS BE SCHEDULED FOR PATIENTS ON MNT?

Follow-up appointments should be scheduled weekly for more serious medical problems requiring medication adjustment as well as for those that choose the 14-day/Phase Plan. Follow-up on a less-frequent basis will be adequate for less-compelling problems and those choosing the 7-day or 3-day/Phase Plans.

### WHAT BRANCHED-CHAIN AMINO ACIDS ARE USED IN PRESCRIPTFIT PRODUCTS?

Although the ratio is a trade secret, the branched-chain and essential amino acids used in the PrescriptFit products include leucine, isoleucine, valine, lysine, histidine, and methionine in proprietary doses.

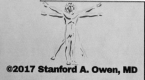

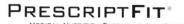

PRESCRIPTFIT
MEDICAL NUTRITION THERAPY ■ ■ ■ ■ ■ ■ ■

# BIBLIOGRAPHY

Amino acids in the 21st Century: The science of amino acid supplements. Report on Amino Acids at ESPEN, Bio Japan 2005. Amino Acids New Link.

Aquilana, R. Oral Amino Acids Administration in Patients with Diabetes Mellitus: Supplementation or Metabolic Therapy? *Am J Cardiol.* 2004 Vol 93(8A), 21-22A

Auguet T, et al. Clinial and adipocytokine changes after bariatric surgery in morbidly obese women. *Obesity.* January 2014; 22(1): 188–194.

Bao Y, et al. Nut consumption inversely associated with mortality. *NEJM.* 2013; 369 (November 21): 2001–2011.

Bazzano, LA et al; Effects of low-carbohydate and low-fat diets. *Annals of Internal Medicine.* 2014; 161: 309–318.

Bray, G. Why do we need drugs to treat the patient with obesity? *Obesity.* 2013; 21(5): 893–899.

Centers for Disease Control and Prevention. National Diabetes Statistics Report: Estimates of Diabetes and Its Burden in the United States. Atlanta, GA: US Department of Health and Human Services. 2014.

Daly M. Relationship of c-reactive protein to obesity-related depressive symptoms: A longitudinal study. *Obesity.* (Jan 2013);
21 (2): 248–250.

The Look AHEAD Research Group. Eight-year weight losses with an intensive lifestyle intervention. *Obesity.* January 2014; 22(1): 5–13.

Feinman, RD. Dietary carbohydrate restriction as the first approach in diabetes management: Critical review and evidence base; *Mayo Clinic Proceedings.* Apri 18, 2014: 1–16.

Feinman, RD; Perspective on fructose. *Nutr Metab* (London). 2013: 9

Forsythe, CE, et al. Comparison of low-fat and low-carbohydrate diets on circulating fatty acid composition and markers of inflammation. *Lipids.* 2008; 43: 65–77.

Fitzpatrick S, et al. Examining behavioral processes through which lifestyle interventions promote weight loss: Results from PREMIER. *Obesity.* April 2014; 22(4): 1002–1007.

Foster, GD, et al. Weight and metabolic outcomes after 2Y on a low-carbohydrate vs. low-fat diet: A randomized trial. *Ann Intern Med.* 2010; 153: 147–157.

Gross, L.S, et al; Increased consumption of refined carbohydrates and the epidemic of type 2 diabetes in the United States: An ecologic assessment. *Am J Clin Nutr.* 2004; 79: 774–779.

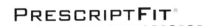

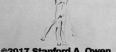

Gudzune, KA, et al. Prior doctor shopping resulting from different treatment correlates with differences in current patient-provider relationships. *Obesity*. Sept 2014; 22(9): 1952–1958.

Guidelines (2013) for managing overweight and obesity in adults. *Obesity*. July 2014; 22(Suppl 2): 401 pages. doi: 10.1002/oby.20818

The Role of Nutritional Supplements with Essential Amino Acids in Patients with Cardiovascular Disease and Diabetes Mellitus, Gheorghiade M, Dioguardi FS, Scognimiglio, R eds. *Am J Cardiol.* 2004; 93(suppl):1A-46A

Hail WL, Milward JF. Casein and Whey eating effects on plasma amino acid profiles, gastrointestinal hormones, and appetite. *Br J Nutr.* 2003; 89:239-248

Hussain, TA, et al; Effect of low-calorie vs. very low calorie ketogenic diet in type 2 diabetes. *Nutrition.* 2012: 28: 1016–1021.

Kaiser Permanente. (2008, July 8). Keeping A Food Diary Doubles Diet Weight Loss, Study Suggests. *ScienceDaily*. Retrieved November 28, 2014 from www.sciencedaily.com/releases/2008/07/080708080738.htm

Landsberg L, et al. Obesity-related hypertension: Pathogenesis, cardiovascular risk, and treatment—A position paper of The Obesity Society and the American Society of Hypertension. *Obesity*. Jan 2013 ; 21(1): 8–24.

Lennerz, B.S., Alsop, D.C., Holsen, L.M., Stein, E., Rojas, R, Ebbeling, C.B., Goldstein, J.M., and Ludwig, D.S. (June 26, 2013). Effects of dietary glycemic index on brain regions related to reward and craving in men. *AmJClin Nutr.* Doi: 10.3945/ajcn.113.064113.

Lent M, et al. Relationship of food addiction to weight loss and attrition during obesity treatment. *Obesity*. January 2014; 22(1): 52–55.

Mattes R, Foster G. Food environment and obesity, A metanalysis review of the literature. *Obesity*. 2014; 22: 2459–2461.

Murak I, et al. Whole fruit, not fruit juice, reduces lifetime risk of type 2 diabetes. *BMJ*. 2013; 347 (August 28): f5001.

National Institutes of Health; National Heart, Lung, and Blood Institute; NHLBI Obesity Education Initiative; and the North American Association for the Study of Obesity. *The Practical Guide.* October 2000; NIH Publication Number 00-4084.

Ninoska, D, et al. Dietary self-monitoring and long-term success with weight management. *Obesity.* Sept 2014; 22(9): 1962–1966.

Pasini E, et al. Amino Acids: Chemistry and Metabolism in Normal and Hypercatabolic States. *Am J Card.* Vol 93(8A), April 2004, 3-5.

Pepino M, et al. Bariatric surgery-induced weight loss causes remission of food addiction in extreme obesity. *Obesity.* August 2014; 22(8): 1792–1798.

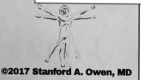

PRESCRIPTFIT®
MEDICAL NUTRITION THERAPY ▪ ▪ ▪ ▪ ▪ ▪ ▪

Puhl R, et al. Obesity bias in training: Attitudes, beliefs, and observations among advanced trainees in professional health disciplines. *Obesity.* April 2014; 22(4): 1008–1015.

Qaseem A, et al. Management of obstructive sleep apnea in adults: A clinical practice guideline from the American College of Physicians. *Ann Int Med.* Oct 1, 2013; 159(7): 471–483.

Rajesh T, et al. Surgical control of diabetes: The role of intestinal vs. gastric mechanisms in the regulation of body weight and glucose homeostasis. *Obesity.* January 2014; 22(1); 159–169.

Reimer, RA. Meat Hydrolysate and essential amino acid-induced GLP-1 secretion is regulated by extracellular signal-regulated kinate1/2 and p38 mitogen-activated protein kinases. *Journal of Endocrinology.* 2006;191:159-170.

Rizza, RA. Pathogenesis of fasting and postprandial hyperglycemia in type 2 diabetes: Implications for therapy. *Diabetes.* 2010; 59: 2697–2707.

Roberts B, et al. Consuming protein with carbohydrate improves glycemic response. *Nutrition.* 2013; 29 (June): 881–885.

Roumie CL, et al. Adding insulin to metformin associated with increased risk of all-cause mortality. *JAMA.* 2014; 311 (June 11): 2288–2296.

Singh M, et al. Weight loss can lead to resolution of GERD symptoms: A prospective intervention trial. *Obesity.* Feb 2013; 21(2): 284–289.

Sin-Tarino PW, et al. Saturated fat, carbohydrate, and cardiovascular disease. *Am J Clin Nur.* 2010; 91: 502–509.

Urban LE, et al. Independent, additive effects of five dietary variables on ad libitum energy intake in a residential study. *Obesity.* September 2014; 22(9): 2018–2024.

Van Der Klaaww A. High protein intake stimulates postprandial GLP1 and PYY release. *Obesity.* August 2013; 21(8); 1602–1607.

Wang, ML, et al. Influence of family, friend and coworker social support and social undermining on weight gain prevention among adults. *Obesity.* Sept 2014 ; 22(9): 1973–1979.

Yang Q, et al. Sugar increases risk of cardiovascular death. *JAMA Int Med.* 2014; February 3: 2012–2015.

Young LH, McNulty PH, et al. Myocardial protein turnover in patients with coronary artery disease: effect of branched chain amino acid infusion. *J Clin Invest.* 1991; 87:554-560

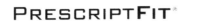

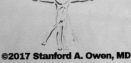

# NOTES

**QUESTIONS?**

EMAIL DR. OWEN AT
DROWENMD@DRDIET.COM

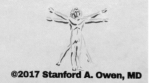

PRESCRIPT**FIT**®

MEDICAL NUTRITION THERAPY

# INDEX

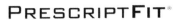

**PRESCRIPTFIT**®
MEDICAL NUTRITION THERAPY ■ ■ ■ ■ ■ ■ ■

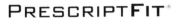

**PRESCRIPTFIT**®
MEDICAL NUTRITION THERAPY ▪ ▪ ▪ ▪ ▪ ▪ ▪

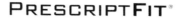

PRESCRIPTFIT
MEDICAL NUTRITION THERAPY

# I

Infertility 202–203
  and cytokines 202
  and MNT 202–203
Inflammation 193, 207–208, 209, 218, 219
Insomnia 204–206, 232
  and cytokines 205
  and MNT 205
  disease/symptom questionnaire 206
Insulin
  and diabetes 8, 14–15, 162
  resistance 7, 8, 14–15, 37, 162–166, 219
  sensitizers 19
Insulin resistance syndrome (IRS) 162
Interleukin 1,2,6,18, 216, 219
Intestinal gas 167
Irritable bowel syndrome (IBS) 167–169, 232
  and cytokines 167
  and MNT 168
  disease/symptom questionnaire 169

# J

Joint pain 72, 207–210, 232
  and cytokines 208
  and MNT 209
  disease/symptom questionnaire 210

# K

Knee pain 208–210
  and cytokines 208
  and MNT 209
  disease/symptom questionnaire 210

# L

Lactose-free 42, 43, 44, 78, 168
LDL 102, 112, 154
Leptin 202, 216, 217, 219
Libido 136

# M

Macrophage inhibiting factor (MIF) 219
Measures 138–139
Medical Nutrition Therapy (MNT) 10–11, 59, 135
  and follow-up appointments 236
  and medication balancing 235
  and physician supervision 138–139, 159, 191
  and quality of life measures 138
  and symptom response 232
  as adjunct treatment 138
  as first-line treatment 138
Medications 18–20. *See also* Pain medications
  and appetite control 229
  and food addiction 18
  and weight loss 229
Metabolic syndrome 162–166
  and cytokines 164
  and MNT 165
  disease/symptom questionnaire 166
Metabolism 63, 70–72, 75, 148, 216
Migraine. *See* Headache
Mood stabilizers 228
Multivitamin 23, 71, 87, 168. *See also* Nutritional supplements
  and compliance 63–64
Muscle fatigue/cramps 211
Muscle tension. *See* Headache

# N

Neuropathy 145, 148
Nutrition
  and beef 114
  and beverages 117–118
  and dairy 120–121
  and eggs 98
  and fruit 103–104
  and nuts 101–102
  and pork 112–113
  and poultry 86–87
  and seafood 81
  and snacks 106–107

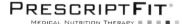

PRESCRIPTFIT®
MEDICAL NUTRITION THERAPY ■ ■ ■ ■ ■ ■ ■ ■    ©2017 Stanford A. Owen, MD

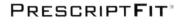

PRESCRIPTFIT
MEDICAL NUTRITION THERAPY ▪ ▪ ▪ ▪ ▪ ▪ ▪

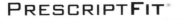

PRESCRIPTFIT®
MEDICAL NUTRITION THERAPY ▪ ▪ ▪ ▪ ▪ ▪ ▪ ▪

# PRODUCTS

AVAILABLE ONLINE AT WWW.DRDIET.COM OR BY CALLING 888-460-6286.

## PrescriptFit™ Shakes, Soups, Puddings

Vanilla

Chocolate

Lactose-Free Vanilla

Lactose-Free Chocolate

Beef

Chicken

## PrescriptFit Snack Bars

Double Chocolate

Toffee

Brownie Bar

Butter Pecan w/ Caramel

Lemon Meringue

Crisp N'Crunch Cinnamon

Crisp N'Crunch Peanut

Crisp N'Crunch Fudge Graham

Chocolate Mint

Oatmeal Cinnamon Raisin

Peanut Butter Crunch

Peanut Butter

Caramel Cocoa

Sweet & Salty Peanut

Crisp N'Crunch Double Berry

Chocolate Almond

## Flavors

Butter Pecan

Mint Chocolate

Orange Cream

Cake Batter

Cinnamon Spice

Chocolate Fudge

Strawberry

Mocha

Black Rasberry

Caramel

Mango

Birthday Cake

## PrescriptFit Educational Material

PrescriptFit Book

PrescriptFit Calendar

The Best Sex Book

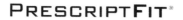

**PRESCRIPTFIT®**

MEDICAL NUTRITION THERAPY